Desi Diet and Health Tips

Desi Diet and Health Tips

South Asian Healthy Cooking

ALI NOOR, MD AND FAZIL ZAFAR

iUniverse, Inc.
Bloomington

Desi Diet and Health Tips
South Asian Healthy Cooking

iUniverse books may be ordered through booksellers or by contacting:

iUniverse
1663 Liberty Drive
Bloomington, IN 47403
www.iuniverse.com
1-800-Authors (1-800-288-4677)

ISBN: 978-1-4620-1970-0 (sc)
ISBN: 978-1-4620-1971-7(dj)
ISBN: 978-1-4620-1972-4(ebk)

Library of Congress Control Number: 2011907504

Printed in the United States of America

iUniverse rev. date: 05/23/2011

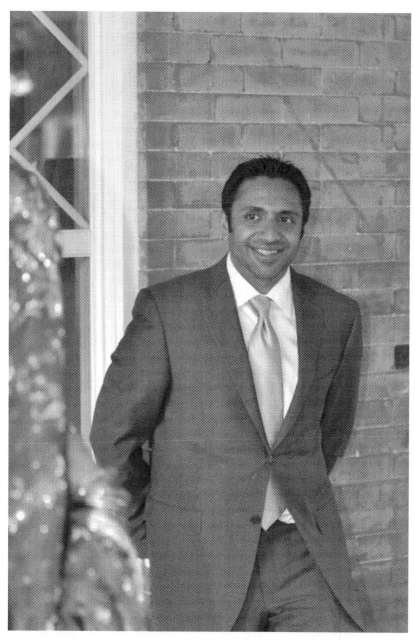

Ali Noor MD

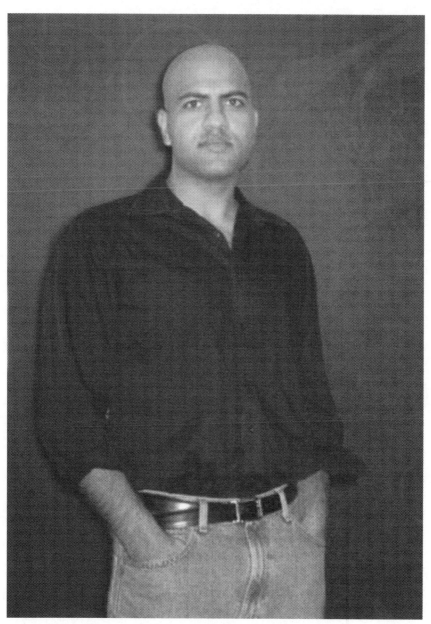

Fazil Zafar

ACKNOWLEDGMENTS

Ali Noor, MD

This book is dedicated to my family for their enthusiasm and support. I am deeply obliged to both my wife, Sadia Arshad Noor, MD, and my mother, Shama Noor, for their help and ideas. I would like to thank my dad, Yacoob Noor, for all his encouragement.I would also like to thank Sumar Hayan, for her help in research and compilation of the data.Last but not the least, I would like to thank my younger brothers, Omar Noor, MD, and Amir Noor, for giving me their precious time and helping to complete the book.

Fazil Zafar

I am deeply indebted to my wife, Tanzeela Zafar, for her support, encouragement, and helping me with ideas in completing this book. I am equally grateful to my Dad Zafar-ul-Islam for his ideas and to my mother Tassawar Islam for her support and encouragement.

CONTENTS

Introduction

If you have grown up Desi, you know how important food is to our culture. Food is a great source of comfort for our people, particularly when we socialize. Many hours are filled by sitting around, from chai (tea) to dinner (and beyond). We spend whole days gossiping, talking, laughing, and eating. It reminds us of our time in our homeland and the loved ones we have there. These foods bring back memories of life back where aromatic spices, delicious meats, and warm, fresh breads made the kitchen table the focal point of our homes and where meals were shared by friends and family in a warm and loving atmosphere.

We had all kinds of different foods, starting with *aam lassi* (or mango lassi), which offsets our spicy foods with its creamy, ever-so-smooth texture. This is followed by kaati roll bites and vada sambar, followed by main courses of hyderabadi chicken biriyani, cabbage with chana daal stir-fry, green beans with cashews, bagaara baingan, dumm aloo, tanddori shrimp tossed with mango, carrots, and red onion salad, cucumbers, and tomato raita. Dinner would follow, with more chai, and of course dessert: warm Qubaani kaa mitha with cool custard or gulaab jamuns and rasgullas. Food was a backdrop *but also central,* and the easy conversation invited all to linger and of course eat some more.

However this familiar scene and these foods we love so much that are so much a part of our heritage make us overeat and may be killing us. A startling 60 percent of all heart disease in the world affects the Desi population. This is a staggering number. Desi or South Asian people, with origins in India, Pakistan, Bangladesh, Nepal, and Sri Lanka, suffer coronary artery disease (CAD) at up to four times the rate of the rest of the planet's population. And unfortunately, conventional screening and treatment do not address the extremely high rates of premature heart attacks among Desis. Many of us suffer heart attacks at an early age, oftentimes without prior symptoms or warning signs. One study among Asian Indian men showed that half of all heart attacks in this population occur under the age of fifty and 25 percent under the age of forty. The worst part is that few physicians in the United States and the subcontinent regularly screen South Asian men and women for these factors prior to a cardiac event.[1]

Our community features an incredibly high incidence of risk factors for coronary artery disease, including insulin resistance, diabetes, a high lipid profile, a generally sedentary lifestyle, and increased, sustained levels of stress. Traditional risk factors do not fully explain the marked increase in the incidence of heart disease among South Asians. These factors seem to go hand in hand with some others that may play a critical role in CAD among the South Asian population. These emerging risk factors include fibrinogen, insulin resistance and metabolic syndrome, low HDL, HDL2b, high triglycerides, small dense LDL, homocysteine, and lipoprotein (a). [2]

How Did Our Culture Get Like This?

Let's face it: in South Asia, there is no concept of health and fitness. South Asians are proud of the ways our culture has been at the vanguard of today's global economy. But even with our global economy changing the world in profound ways every day, our culture's concern for basic health and fitness is woefully inadequate.

Think back to your mother's pantry in your childhood home. Can you remember *any* food that actually came with a nutrition label? Of course not; but we happily ate anything and everything, with little concern for what was actually going into our bodies. We would eat tons of food filled with *gee* (one of the worst types of fat), not to mention the constant supply of *roti* and *paratha* (breads) slathered in butter. But of course, it would be too easy to just blame everything on our parents and our culture at large.

Generally, no matter where in the world we live, there are several principal reasons that people develop unhealthy eating habits. The first reason is too few meals during the day. When we go on a diet, we tend to skip meals—particularly breakfast. However, these meals we skip early in the day add up in bad ways. They result in an overwhelming temptation to eat more later in the day. Skip breakfast, and you may find yourself stuffing your face with roti and paratha later—or worse yet, standing in line at a fast food restaurant.

Being unaware of calories and fat is a second disturbing principle. Most of us eat with no regard to the caloric and/or fat content of the foods we ingest. This can lead to weight gain and increased unhealthy eating habits. It is not difficult to eat one-and-a-half or even twice the normal calories required to maintain your weight if you have no idea how many calories you are eating.

Unfortunately, junk food leads to more junk food. As you probably already know, eating unhealthy food makes you crave even more unhealthy food. A handful of chips, for example, will leave you wanting another handful, and so on. ("Betcha can't eat just one" was the slogan for one chip brand, in fact, for good reason.)

American society has finally started to understand the negative effects of poor eating habits; increased attention is being paid to better eating and more reasonable portion sizes. For example, many areas are now mandating that restaurants post the calorie content of all their menu items. Additionally, more and more low-calorie and low-fat options are available both in our supermarkets and restaurants that were not around even a decade ago. Additionally, our public school students are given healthier meal options. Wide now have several 24/7 cable food channels (with many of the programs focusing on healthy cooking), and nutritionists are sprouting up everywhere.

Unfortunately, our Desi population lags behind in both proper nutrition and exercise. Some have faced challenges adapting to the food and culture; the lifestyle is so different they are not sure how to adjust. I work as a fitness trainer in New York, and I joke that I can always spot the Desi. Typically, they seem oddly perplexed by even basic workout equipment. However, this scene reflects a more serious problem, one that comes down to our basic beliefs about the value of exercise and nutrition.

Why Is Food So Important to Our Health?

Sure, we have known for ages that eating too much will make us gain weight. More recently, one scientific study after the other has proved that obesity is linked to many diseases, including heart disease, stroke, diabetes, several types of cancer, sleep apnea, osteoarthritis, gout, gallbladder-related diseases, and others. However, over the past two decades, a scientific revolution, the mapping of our genes has helped us to better understand the dynamic impact that food has on our bodies. This new science, termed nutrigenomics—the science of how food talks to your genes—can lead to incredible health benefits.

Nutrigenomics is not about finding the perfect diet. We used to assume that our genetic code simply sat around practically useless in storage in our cells until we passed it on to our offspring. However, this genomic revolution has opened up an entirely new world of understanding about what our genes really do. Of course, genes do control our physical characteristics, but that is only a small bit of it. Our genes actually control all of the daily flow of instructions that regulates every aspect of our biochemistry and physiology, controlling hormone production, brain messenger chemicals, blood pressure, and cholesterol, not to mention our moods and aging processes. It also controls our risk of acquiring conditions like heart disease and cancer. Not surprisingly, our genes play a particularly important role in controlling our metabolism and weight.

Perhaps the most important part of these breakthroughs is that nutrigenomics has improved our understanding of both food and calories. We now know that food contains hidden information communicated to our genes, giving our metabolism specific instructions on what it should be doing, from losing weight to gaining weight, increasing or decreasing cholesterol, and producing molecules that directly affect our appetites.

Armed with this knowledge, it is now possible to lose weight, keep it off, and increase our overall health with a minimum of "work." This new knowledge is incredibly powerful, so much so that when our body has a condition where it is not functioning correctly, we can harness the powers of better nutrition to minimize the problem. And it is with this knowledge that we created the Desi Diet.

Introducing . . . the Desi Diet

In creating the Desi Diet, we focused on simplicity and ease-of-use. We have found a way for you to lose weight for the long-term, increase your overall health, and look and feel better without obsessing over calories and eating foods you hate. Simplicity is key; actually, at the core of the Desi Diet are two basic ideas:

- In traditional Desi culture, we eat large dinners and almost no breakfast. In the *Desi Diet* book, breakfast is the most important meal.

- In traditional Desi culture, everything is cooked in saturated fat. In the *Desi Diet* book, we cook with polyunsaturated fat (a "good fat" that can be found in fish, nuts, seeds, and vegetable oils, including soybean, corn, safflower, canola, olive, and sunflower oils.)

There's more to it than that, of course. However, you'll still be able to enjoy your *roti* and *paratha*, just without all that ghee. You'll even get to eat your kaati rolls and vada sambar, hyderabadi chicken biriyani, or tandori shrimp. However, instead, we will focus on cooking the foods we love with healthier methods, reducing our portion sizes and eating more often, and even getting out there and doing some exercise.

Why We Wrote This Book

While I joke about my fellow Desis at the gym, our culture's health neglect is a particularly personal and serious matter to me. My father, who suffered a heart attack, currently is fighting diabetes. Of my two uncles, one died from a heart attack; the other died from diabetes. Unfortunately, from what I have seen, these scenarios aren't confined to the older generations. As my social circle of Desi friends gets older, I notice that they become unhealthier with each passing year. I have dedicated my life to healthy living, and I realize that it is important to get the word out to our community now so that our future generations can benefit.

My partner in creating the *Desi Diet*, Dr. Ali Noor, MD, has similar motivations. His father had a bypass at the age of forty-seven. Growing up in this culture, eating the same types of foods, and avoiding exercise led Ali to the point where he was nearly sixty pounds overweight. However, looking at his own father and seeing himself in the not-too-distant future, he began to worry about his future health and realized he needed to change his ways. He committed to the plan presented here; to date, he has lost almost sixty pounds, changing his life and his future health.

As a physician and growing up in the Desi culture, Dr. Noor feels as though it is his responsibility to help the people he grew up with and help the Desi population as a whole with their current and future health because the population is lagging so far behind our American counterparts when it comes to nutrition and exercise and more importantly, because we are losing so many of our loved ones at such early ages.

Last, I feel it is important to educate the community now so that our future generations can benefit. And for a purely selfish reason, I want to do this for my own daughter.

How to Use This Book

You will find this book to be enjoyable to read and easy to use. It will give you a clear, simple path to follow that you can start today and immediately begin seeing results.

You can read it straight through from beginning to end or concentrate on areas that are of particular interest to you. Two things are certain: you'll definitely want to come back to certain sections again and again, and you'll be surprised how downright delicious and healthy the cuisine of our homeland can be.

With the *Desi Diet*, you will take a proactive role in determining your own health. The changes recommended can be implemented gradually and without a lot of the resistance common in the typical "yo-yo diet." If you have questions on specific food types, like proteins, carbs, or fats, and their roles in the body, you will find that information throughout the book. If you are interested in simple lifestyle changes that have nothing to do with food, such as vitamins and minerals and their role in the body, how to better manage your water intake for optimal health, or the importance of sleeping, these each have their own chapter as well.

This book also includes plenty of menus, from the perfect dish to easy-to-find ingredients, even if you live in a small town. The *Desi Diet* comes complete with recipes for delicious, easy-to-prepare meals as well. We even provide convenient shopping lists that will provide you with all the foods (complete with nutrition labels, of course) that you will need for an entire week, as well as simple, on-the-go snack foods. There are recommendations on vitamins and supplements, better sleeping habits, and much more. The best part of this book? You can implement it at your own pace. There are no strict diets to follow, and you certainly won't have to obsess about counting calories. The secret is, by using the principles of nutrigenomics, if you follow even some of the advice in this book, weight will begin to come off—even without you "trying" to lose weight.

The Secret about the Desi Diet

Although we titled this book *Desi Diet*, it is about much more than a diet: it's about making a lifestyle change.

In fact, study after study has proven that most (nearly 95 percent.) of diets do not work. Instead, most dieters actually go on to gain weight once the diet period is over. However, the lifestyle change presented in *Desi Diet* will bring you better health and a more enjoyable, longer life. Although it is written for people from South Asia, anyone can use it. We show you how and why to live a healthy lifestyle—including proper sleeping habits, when to eat, controlling portion sizes, better cooking methods, and more—all things that will boost your long-term health.

Since a young age, I have trained in Shaolin Kung Fu. I can remember to this day the words of my teacher, who would tell me, "This is not a hobby, this is a lifestyle; if you live it then you will be it." That has been my inspiration, and I feel it applies to everything in this book as well. I can speak as a physical trainer, regarding my clients—and for Dr. Noor, as a physician with his patients—we have never told anyone, once, to "lose weight." We have asked them to better understand their bodies and eating habits and not fight against them. This is what is possible with the *Desi Diet*, and we believe it will work for you, too.

Proteins, Carbohydrates, and Fats

Proteins, carbohydrates, and fats make up the three major, or macro, nutrients. Although they are each required by the body for healthy living, they are each very different and thus, must be consumed differently for optimal health. This chapter will tell you the important points you need to know about each. Along the way, we'll shatter some common myths about each and show you how to eat them and when to eat them. Most importantly, after reading this chapter, you will know how to incorporate each into the *Desi Diet*.

Proteins

Protein is absolutely essential for cell maintenance and repair and regulates a wide range of our bodies' functions. Proteins account for the bulk of cell structure; some function as enzymes and catalyze cellular activities. One key point to know is that how much protein we need to eat each day depends on our ideal body weight. This is because amino acids are not needed by fat cells, only by our lean body mass. Unlike carbohydrates and fats, proteins are comprised of a nitrogen-containing group called amino acids.

These amino acids function exactly like building blocks. There are twenty-two amino acids, and they are divided into two main categories: Indispensable Amino Acids (IAAs) and Dispensable Amino Acids (DAAs). Essential amino acids must appear in our diet because they are not and cannot be made by the body. The eight essential amino acids are: isoleucine, leucine, lysine, methionine, phenylalanine, threonine, tryptophan, and valine.

Although we don't think about it when we eat our turkey sandwich for lunch or chicken marsala for dinner, the content and balance of amino acids—and most importantly the ratio of IAA to DAA—determines the health-maintaining value of a protein.

The Three Categories of Protein

Proteins can be broken into three main categories, depending on the speed in which they are broken down by our bodies: 1. fast-absorbing, 2. medium-absorbing, and 3. slow-absorbing. As far as our natural food sources go, fish, chicken, meat, and eggs provide great fast-absorbing protein; dairy products provide slow-absorbing proteins.

Tips to remember regarding protein consumption:

- **Take fast-absorbing proteins first thing in the morning and after workouts** since the body needs these immediately in order to prevent muscle breakdown. (When we exercise, our muscles naturally look for amino acids/proteins to rebuild muscle.)
- **Muscle burns more calories than fat,** so if you lose muscle, you burn fewer calories per pound of body weight. And this is exactly why many people who go on restricted-calorie diets find they have problems losing fat and become flabby and bloated.
- **Take slow proteins before traveling or when you will be without proteins for awhile.** Slow proteins, such as casein from milk, are good when you will be without nourishment for hours. This way, protein breaks down slowly, slowing muscle loss, even though you are not eating.
- **Don't forget turkey!** In Desi culture, we do not eat a lot of turkey, since the bird is not native to our homelands. However, turkey is an excellent source of L-tryptophan, which later converts to the 5HTP amino acid and also suppresses cortisol levels. Cortisol is one of the main causes for excess fat storage and can lead to many age-related diseases.

On a personal note, when I visit Pakistan, I don't have access to protein shakes, so every morning I eat four eggs and then work out on the rooftop lifting bricks as my weights. (We told you health and fitness is a lagging concept in the Southern Asia!) It is very hot there, so I do my workout very early in the morning. Afterward, I usually eat *keema* (cooked ground meat). My aunt finds this weird, since this is typically a dinnertime meal. Additionally, I usually drink *laasi* immediately before hiking. The sugar provides energy, while the casein protein prevents muscle breakdown while outdoors for hours without a meal.

On my recent trips to this area, I have noticed a recent trend that might be due to Bollywood movies: more and more Desis seem to be trying to build up their bodies. However, they seem be going about it in the wrong way, thinking that if they keep eating *roti,* they will gain muscle. However, *roti* does not provide a good source of protein. This protein-*roti* myth might have risen because back in the day someone would eat a few *roties* and be able to walk miles without getting tired. However, this energy was because of the food's carbohydrate content, not protein. However, people have taken this myth too far. People eat a few *roties* and don't really work it off, adding useless, unused calories to their daily intake, which later converts to fat.

Carbohydrates

Simply put, carbohydrates, or "carbs," are sugars that provide our body with energy. However, you will see that all carbs are not created equally. Consuming "good" carbs can help transform our bodies into lean, fat-burning machines; eating too many "bad" carbs can be as detrimental to our overall health as any junk food.

Good Carbs and Their Benefits

"Good carbs" (or "complex carbs") are carbohydrates that are still in, or at least close to, their natural state. These are "whole foods" that have not been processed or otherwise altered by humans or our machines. These carbs are generally high in fiber and give our bodies energy over sustained periods of time—and contribute to a sense of "feeling full." Besides all these health benefits, good carbs lower cholesterol levels and help our bodies eliminate toxins.

Good carbs also have something called a low glycemic index (GI). It is important to know that foods with a low glycemic index will not spike our blood sugar (important for all of us; critical for diabetics.) Additionally, good carbs are nutritious, and they contain many vitamins, minerals, and other nutrients.

Good Carbs Include:

- Fruits

- Vegetables
- Beans
- Legumes
- Nuts
- Seeds
- Whole grain breads, cereals, pastas
- Milk, cottage cheese

Bad Carbs

Bad carbs are those foods that have been refined and processed and are not as they occur in nature. A good example of this is white bread. This refining and processing has removed most of their nutritional value, replacing them with excessive additives, such as colorings, flavorings, and preservatives.

The problem with bad carbs is that they are everywhere. They are, admittedly, very tasty. They are packaged (and marketed!) for our on-the-go lifestyle. Yet, they are extremely unhealthy for us, because they aren't easily digested and tend to spike our blood sugar levels. Unfortunately, these foods consist of a good part of most Desi and American diets and include: candy, snacks, baked goods (with refined white flour), white pastas, sodas, and many other common foods and beverages.

Eat an excess of bad carbs and you will gain weight. These foods are laden with "empty calories" (i.e., having no nutritional value). Bad carbs are a huge factor in the many diseases plaguing our society, from diabetes to metabolic syndrome and heart disease to obesity, to name just a few. And although eating bad carbs will give us an energy boost (in reality, just a "spike"), the energy quickly dissipates, making us feel hungry all over again and thus craving more carbs—starting this bad cycle all over again.

We cannot overstate the importance of good carbs enough. Just some of their benefits include:

- *Good carbs aid weight management.* Not surprisingly, good carbs (i.e., high in complex carbohydrates) are usually lower in calories. Thus, it will take more time to eat two hundred calories of fresh apple than it will to eat two hundred calories of chocolate cake. And on a calorie-for-calorie basis, good carbs are more satisfying and add up more slowly than bad carbs.

- *Good carbs contain fiber, which keeps us feeling full longer.* The majority of us don't consume the recommended amounts of fiber per day (thirty-eight grams for men and twenty-five grams for women under the age of fifty). By eating more good carbs, we also are consuming more fiber, thus cutting down on the overall amount of food we eat.
- *They are filled with great nutrients.* Good carbs are loaded with *vitamins*, minerals, phytochemicals, and other nutrients that just aren't present in bad carbs.

Sticking to a Good-Carb Diet

While Americans have never been more interested in good carbs, trying to follow a good-carb diet is not without its potential pitfalls. Some food manufacturers have been taking advantage of this burgeoning interest with multiple ways to confuse those seeking good/complex carbs.

For example, the regulation on much of food labeling is very weak and not entirely clear. Any food with even a miniscule amount of whole grain can be called a "whole grain." Always examine the labels of "whole grain foods." Anything that is "enriched" is highly-processed and contains no significant amount of whole grain. Likewise, many specious claims are made about fiber. A decent serving of whole grains will have at least three grams of fiber. Only pick cereals, pastas, grains, and breads that meet this amount.

Last, remember that you can never go wrong eating fresh fruit and vegetables. They are the best available source of good carbs, loaded with nutrients—and fiber—and are the perfect snack at just about any time of the day.

Fats

As recently as a few decades ago, the prevailing mantra was that if we eliminate the fats from our diets, we could eliminate the fat from our bodies. These days, however, we know better. Just as with carbs, there are good fats and then there are bad fats. In fact, fats are a critical part of the human diet—and one of the three mega-nutrients. Fats provide a myriad of health benefits: they deliver essential fatty acids, provide fat-soluble vitamins, maintain the softness of our skin, and energize our entire body. In fact, the US Department of Agriculture recommends in its dietary guidelines that adults obtain 20 percent to 35 percent of their calories consumed from fats. And at a bare minimum, we must gather at least 10 percent of our total caloric intake from fat.

However, the grave problem is that the average American obtains 34 percent to 40 percent of our calories from fat. While Desis may have less fat in their diets, the fats we do eat tend to be the unhealthy trans—and saturated-fat varieties. Why are fats so widely popular across cultures and continents? Simple enough: fats taste good and are present in much of the processed food clogging our diets.

Fats Aren't the Only Things Making Us Fat

Fat is made out to be the enemy in many diets, but actually, fats present many life-affirming health benefits. Fats supply essential fatty acids (EFAs). Since our bodies are unable to produce EFAs (such as linoleic acid and alpha-linolenic acid), we must find them in food. Fat is also the "driver" for essential vitamins A, D, E, and K (known as fat-soluble vitamins) into and around our bodies. Fat is also critical for keeping our skin healthy and helps promote proper eyesight and brain development in babies and kids.

As we mentioned, fats—perhaps counter-intuitively—are not the only thing making us obese, and eating fats does not make us fat. Obesity is caused by overeating more than just any one nutrient. Fats are critical to our diets, and some fats make us healthier. Eating more calories—whether from fats, carbs, or proteins—than we burn off each day will lead to weight gain. Not enough exercise and too much food (even healthier foods) will make us fat. Additionally, our genetics, age, sex, and overall lifestyle factor in here, too.

That's the good news. The truth is, fats still do play a sizeable role in our obesity epidemic. With nine calories per gram, fats are calorie-dense; carbs and protein have only four calories per gram, in comparison. And it's easy to eat too many fats because they loom in just about everything our culture offers: from French fries to steaks; cakes to processed breads; all kinds of sweets to just about anything that can be canned, processed, or otherwise refined. Unfortunately, eating too many of the bad fats does more than make our favorite pair of jeans a little tight. Our cultures' (yes, that's an American and Desi thing) obsession with the wrong kinds of fats has caused a rise in all kinds of diseases, including type-2 diabetes, morbid obesity, heart disease, and others. Eating fewer fats (to an extent) and eating the right kinds of fats helps us lose weight, and in the process, decreases our risk for developing life-threatening illnesses.

Good—and Bad—Fats

In general, there are two groups of fats: saturated and unsaturated. Each group is broken down into several others. We'll first investigate the good kind of fats: unsaturated.

Unsaturated fats include polyunsaturated fatty acids and monounsaturated fats. Each type, when eaten in moderation, and when replacing saturated or trans fats, will lower cholesterol levels and reduce our risk of heart disease.

Polyunsaturated fats are found predominantly in vegetable oils. These help lower both blood cholesterol and triglyceride levels, particularly when replacing saturated fats. One type of polyunsaturated fat receiving a lot of attention lately for its heart-health properties is omega-3 fatty acid. Omega-3s are found in both fatty fish (like salmon, trout, catfish, and mackerel), walnuts, and flaxseed. Fish contain the most effective "long-chain" type of omega-3s; the American Heart Association recommends that we eat two servings of these fatty fish per week. (However, remember that positive benefits of eating fish can be canceled by the poor effects that come with frying it in saturated fats!)

Monounsaturated fats are the other "good" unsaturated fat. They have been found to reduce the chances of developing heart disease. Mediterranean countries consume lots of these, primarily as olive oil. Known as the "Mediterranean diet," these countries are renowned for having low levels of heart disease. Typically found in liquid form at room temperature, monounsaturated fats solidify when refrigerated. These fats contain ample supplies of the antioxidant vitamin E, a heart-healthy nutrient that is often missing from American and Desi diets. These fats are found in olives, avocados, nuts (hazelnuts, almonds, Brazil nuts, cashews), seeds (sesame and pumpkin), and oils (olive, canola, and peanut).

Bad Fats Are Everywhere

Saturated fats and trans fatty acids are two fat types that raise cholesterol, clog arteries, and increase heart disease risk. Of course, they should be eaten sparingly. Saturated fats commonly occur in animal products (meat, poultry skin, high-fat dairy, eggs, etc.) and room-temperature liquid vegetable fats, like coconut and palm oils. Saturated fats should be limited to just 7 to 10 percent of our total fat calories, at most.

When eaten excessively, saturated fat can cause blocked arteries, increasing the risk of heart attack and stroke. Saturated fat is worse than even dietary cholesterol, as it relates to raising blood cholesterol levels, a risk factor for both heart disease and stroke. Actually, there is no dietary requirement for saturated fat because our bodies produce all that it needs. However, as we mentioned, there is no need to completely avoid foods with saturated fat for good health; foods like meat, cheese, and milk pack a multitude of nutrients, including protein, vitamins, and minerals. As long as we keep saturated fat to less than 7 percent of all the fat we eat, we are okay.

Trans fatty acids, or "trans fats," are everywhere today, least of which is in the news. Trans fats are further divided into two types: naturally occurring (found in trace amounts in dairy and meat products) and artificial (when liquid oils are hardened into partially-hydrogenated fats). Fortunately, natural trans fats are not a problem, particularly when eating low-fat dairy or lean meat products. The real culprit in American diets—and even more so in Desi culture—are artificial trans fats. These partially hydrogenated oils are pervasive in fried foods, baked goods (like cookies, icings, crackers, packaged snack foods), microwave popcorn, some margarines, fast foods, and sorry, just about every traditional Desi recipe that calls for frying. Lately, physicians and researchers have determined that trans fats are even worse for our bodies than saturated fats, even butter or lard.

Trans fats are so bad because they act as a direct assault on our heart-health. Even minor amounts of artificial trans fats increase the risk for heart disease by increasing LDL (bad) cholesterol and decreasing HDL (good) cholesterol. Today, most health organizations urge us to keep trans fat consumption (even the less-troublesome natural variety) to as little as possible. The Harvard School of Public Health has estimated that eliminating trans fats from the American diet could prevent about two hundred and fifty thousand heart attacks yearly (imagine what it could do for Desi culture!) In the United States, partially hydrogenated fat (trans fat) is gradually being removed from most packaged foods. But it's still found in some stick margarine, shortening, fast food, cookies, crackers, granola bars, and microwave popcorn. And in our Desi culture, no one really knows how prevalent trans fat is, because the quality of food labeling is so poor.

An Easy Guide to Keeping Your Fats Straight

Adding to the confusion surrounding which fats are good and which are bad is the way in which we classify them. Most foods, in fact, are made up of several types of fats. However, fats are typically classified according to whichever fat is dominant in their makeup. Examples of the different types of fats include:

Saturated Fats/Trans Fatty Acids/Polyunsaturated Monounsaturated Fats

Butter	Corn oil	Canola oil
Lard	Fish oil	Almond oil
Lunchmeat and Meat	Soybean oil	Walnut oil
Poultry (and skin)	Safflower oil	Olive oil
Coconut products	Sesame oil	Peanut oil
Palm/palm kernel oil and products	Cottonseed oil	Avocado
Dairy products (not skim milk)	Sunflower oil	Olives
Partially hydrogenated oils	Nuts and seeds	Peanut butter

Know Your Fats—and Read Your Labels

The only way to truly know your fat consumption is to know your fats (illustrated in the chart above) and to become a label reader. On your food's nutrition facts panel, you can find all needed information required to make better, healthier food choices. Always look for foods low in total fat—and particularly in saturated and trans fats.

Beware the "trans fat trap": Because of loopholes in our food labeling regulations, manufacturers are allowed to call their food "trans fat free" or the even more misleading "0 grams trans fat" and still have up to ½ gram—not per container, but per serving! Needless to say, these can add up quickly.

The following tips will also help you reduce the total amount of fat in your diet:

- Eat plenty of whole grains, fruits, and vegetables every day.
- Try to eat one vegetarian meal—with plenty of beans—at least once weekly.

- Choose dairy products that are low-fat or skim.
- Try reduced-fat salad dressings (that don't have an overabundance of sugars).
- Switch from fat-laden sauces to vinegars, mustards, and lemon juice.
- Eat the right fats: try unsaturated liquid oils (like canola or olive) and ditch the butter or partially-hydrogenated margarine.
- Cut down on high-fat foods, like processed or fried foods, sweets, and desserts.
- When cooking at home, choose the lower-fat alternative (like low-fat cream cheese) when possible.

Fat in My Diet: What's Right for Me?

When examining food labels for fat content, it is important to know your daily fat allowance. Doing so will help you better understand how a serving of that food fits into your diet. Following are some examples of healthy daily fat allowances:

1,800 calories per day

- Forty to seventy grams of total fat
- Fourteen grams or less of saturated fat
- Two grams or less of trans fat

2,200 calories per day

- Forty-nine to eight-six grams of total fat
- Seventeen grams or less of saturated fat
- Three grams or less of trans fat

2,500 calories per day

- Fifty-six to ninety-seven grams of total fat
- Twenty grams or less of saturated fat
- Three grams or less of trans fat

The Bottom Line on Fats

Always try to choose healthy fats, eat less saturated fats, limit saturated fat, and avoid trans fat.

What's important to remember is that the total amount of fat we eat isn't directly correlated with disease. What is truly of importance is the *type of fat* we eat. Bad fats—trans fats and saturated fats—increase risk for disease. Good fats—monounsaturated and polyunsaturated fats—lower disease risk. Although it is important to limit cholesterol intake (particularly if you suffer from diabetes or heart disease), dietary cholesterol is not nearly as bad for us as it has been portrayed.

The biggest influence on blood cholesterol level is the mix of fats in our diets—not the amount of cholesterol we get from food.

Conclusion

Always remember that moderation and balance is critical. Balancing carbs, proteins, and fat is key. In short, remember to:

- Keep carbohydrates to a maximum of 40 percent of your daily calories
- Make sure at least half of your grains are whole grains
- Eat five servings of fruit and vegetables per day

In the beginning, stick to the rules above, try some of the great foods listed in our chapter on recipes, and you'll be on your way to losing weight naturally, feeling better, and improving your overall health.

Calories—and Their Importance to Your Diet

Calories and counting them are an important part of weight and fat loss. But what are calories, exactly? Scientifically speaking, a calorie is the quantity of heat required to raise the temperature of one gram of water one degree Celsius from a standard initial temperature. For the purpose of *Desi Diet* as well as the standard unit of measure in nutrition, a calorie may be defined as a unit of energy-producing potential equal to the quantity of heat contained in food and released upon oxidation by the body. A food's caloric content depends on its nutrient content and can include carbohydrates, fats, and proteins. These three main nutrients (or mega-nutrients) are released during digestion and then absorbed into our bodies' bloodstream and converted into glucose or blood sugar. Energy from food that is not needed immediately can be stored as body fat, and these energy stores can be used by the body later on.

Although calories are important, there are two caveats that we will repeat time and time again throughout this book:

- Counting calories is important to fat and weight loss, but especially so when paired with a proper nutritional plan and some form of physical activity.
- All calories are not the same. One hundred calories of nutrient-rich fruits or vegetables are more beneficial than one hundred calories of soda, for example.

Fat and weight loss are all about cutting the ratio between calories in versus calories out: when you cut your calorie consumption and exercise, your body will lose fat and excess weight. And to maintain this healthy weight range, you must balance the calories (from food and drinks) with calories expanded. The number of calories we eat directly impacts our metabolism, which is why, as we decrease the number of overall calories, it becomes especially important to eat the right calories. Cutting back on "empty" calories lacking nutrients and vitamins is smart; cutting nutrient-rich foods blindly will hurt your body in the long run. The *Desi Diet* is filled with ideas on making wiser food choices. This will help you cut calories naturally, lose weight, and still allow you the freedom to enjoy some of the foods you love so much.

Study after study has found that the optimal approach is to cut fewer calories and increase our activity levels. If we just cut calories, and avoid exercise altogether, our bodies will lose lean body mass and tissue, because (as we will discuss in-depth later), when our bodies sense that we are starving ourselves, our brain believes that we are going into "starvation" mode, and thus holds onto body fat. Instead, if we increase our physical activity, our metabolism will increase naturally, burning energy and removing some of our stored fat and reserves to burn fat and help gain muscle.

Rethinking Weight Loss

There is a problem inherent in all restrictive-calorie diets (and most diets do restrict calories): they don't recognize that calorie consumption actually increases our bodies' metabolism, therefore helping us to lose weight. If we consider calories this way, a striking paradigm emerges:

Since our bodies require a constant energy supply to stay alive, consuming calories is a way of eating ourselves thin not starving ourselves thin.

We know that the majority of Americans and Desis are heading toward obesity. Yes, reducing calories will help cut fat loss, but only to a point. To really lose the optimal amounts of fat and weight and keep them off, we need to eat fewer calories, increase our physical activity, and make better (i.e., healthier) food choices.

Finding Our Optimal Calorie Intake

Each of us has a recommended daily calorie intake. Finding your own is paramount in any successful weight loss plan. By finding our base amount, we can understand where our current diet is—and what excess "empty-calorie" foods can be easily eliminated. This recommended calorie intake also considers our gender, age, height, and activity levels. For example, a six-foot tall, lean, thirty-year-old man will have a different caloric requirement than a five-foot tall, stout, forty-year-old woman. There are two key factors in determining the amount of calories we need to consume each day, or total calories needed (TCN): *1) our basal metabolic rate (BMR) and 2) our activity level.*

BMR, or basal metabolic rate, is the minimum number of calories (i.e., energy) needed by our body to complete basic, involuntary functions like our heartbeat, breathing, heat generation, and production and transmission of neuroendocrine signals required for everyday body processes. Our BMR is directly responsible for the consumption of about 60 percent to 70 percent of the total calories our body uses. Exercise (physical activity) accounts for approximately 30 percent; digestion and absorption require the remaining 10 percent of total calories consumed.

There are a myriad of different factors influencing our BMR: age, body size/composition, genetics, gender, environmental temperature, overall calorie consumption and diet, our body's physical condition, and our total activity level. Age is particularly important. From childhood to our young adult years, the body has incredibly high energy demands as we are continually building up bone, muscle, and tissue. In fact, during our infancy, our bodies have the highest demand and our energy need per pound is at the highest level of our entire lifetime. (Which is exactly why so many of us get to college, continue our old eating habits as our bodies' metabolism starts to slow down, and we end up packing on the "freshman fifteen.")

Our BMR decreases as we age. For every ten years that we age, our required energy drops approximately 2 percent. So, then, a man aged twenty-five may need to consume 2,200 calories each day—but by the age of thirty-five, that same man will need only 2,100 calories, and the numbers decrease from here. The only way to maintain a level BMR and energy need is to practice a steady level of physical activity throughout your life.

Our body sizes and composition also impact our energy needs. All of our bodies consist of lean tissue, muscle, bone, and fat. Since muscle burns more energy than body fat, the higher the ratio of muscle to fat, the more calories we need to maintain any given body weight. Regarding body composition, a person with a muscular, athletic frame has a higher metabolism than a person with a fatty, heavier frame. Therefore, by increasing muscle and decreasing our bodies fat, we increase our BMR. Our body types also directly affects the amount of energy our bodies needs. For example, a thin, tall body has more surface area than a short body: this means that in the thinner, taller individual, more heat is lost and likewise, the more calories are required to be burned to maintain normal body temperature. When body fat percentage is lower, our BMR is higher.

Genetics and family history are aspects of our makeup that affect BMR, and unfortunately, cannot be changed. We do tend to pick up eating habits from our parents and older siblings, which is some of the reason why family members often have the same body weight and type. However, a much greater impact is from our genetics. They play a tremendous role in what sort of metabolism we have.

BMR is influenced by gender, too. Because men have a lower percentage of body fat and higher level of muscle mass, they generally have a higher metabolism than their female counterparts. Through their adult years, men will have anywhere from 10 percent to 20 percent more muscle (and less body fat) than women of the same height and age. Men's basic energy needs are fundamentally higher due to muscle building. Overall, men have a lower body fat percentage than women, hence the reason why men have a 10 percent to 15 percent higher BMR than women. Women naturally keep a certain amount of body fat stored—in preparation for a possible pregnancy (and breastfeeding). This is why during pregnancy, and immediately following it, the energy a woman needs increases (and thus, so does her caloric intake). Because of the demands of pregnancy, a woman may have to eat upwards of an additional three hundred calories per day. This adds up pretty quickly: three hundred extra calories per day is an additional eighty thousand-plus calories over the course of an average nine-month pregnancy! Once she gives birth, she is not off the hook either: breastfeeding raises this caloric need even further, to a total of five hundred extra calories per day, for the average lactating woman.

Environmental temperature also impacts BMR. When the outside temperature drops, your body must burn more calories to keep it warm. Thus, your BMR revs slightly higher when it is exposed for any length of time to cold temperatures. This is especially so if your body gets so cold that you shiver or move around to keep warm. In general, extreme temperatures cold or hot require increased calories, because of the shock associated with keeping the body's metabolic activities balanced.

The greatest impact on BMR is, of course, caloric consumption. The connection is so strong, in fact, that if you were to starve yourself, your BMR can immediately drop as much as 30 percent; some extreme calorie restrictive diets can drop BMR up to 20 percent. However, this is not beneficial either for your health, or your weight-loss goals:

Drastically cutting calories or starving yourself is unhealthy and may actually make it more difficult for you to lose weight.
Severe drops in BMR will force your body to go into survival or "starvation" mode, dramatically decreasing metabolic processes so much so that the body actually hangs onto its body fat stores.

Remember that movement in any form, whether going to bed at night to sprinting around a track, is physical energy, and thus, requires energy. For most people, physical energy (yes, even down to blinking your eyes) makes up approximately 30 percent of your body's caloric/energy need. (For active people, this number can be up to 40 percent of our total energy.) The type, intensity, and length of the physical activity will determine the amount of calories and energy it will burn. The FDA suggests that you do approximately five hours of moderately intense physical activity per week to lose excess body fat. Besides weight loss, exercise carries a plethora of health benefits as well. The reduced weight has been proven to lower risk for stroke, type-2 diabetes, high blood pressure, and heart disease. Repeated studies have shown that ongoing exercise can create better mental well-being, too.

As BMR is influenced by body type and size, so is the energy needed to complete any physical activity: it takes more energy for a 250 lb person to run around the block than it does for someone who weighs 125 lbs. For example, a brisk, 30-minute walk burns about 155 calories in a 120 lb person, but only 110 calories in a 100 lb person. This relation between body size and energy is yet another factor in why men can more easily burn calories than women: men typically weigh more than women. When you consider how even moderate physical activities can have a profound impact on calories burned, you see its importance in any healthy living plan: for a 150 lb person, even golfing or biking can burn approximately 300 calories per hour. Not surprisingly, more intensive activities are perfect choices for an exercise plan; moderate jogging or bicycling can burn 600 calories per hour in that same 150 lb person.

How to Determine your Total Calorie Needs (TCN)

Our calorie needs are based on two different numbers: our basal metabolic rate (BMR) and our activity level. In other words, our total calorie needs (TCN) equals our BMR x an allowance for our activity levels, called the Activity Multiplier. Obtaining the two parts to our equation:

BMR

BMR is best represented by a formula called the Harris-Benedict formula, and is different for men and women:

Men: 66 + (13.7 x wt in kg) + (5 x ht in cm) – (6.8 x age in years)
Women: 655 + (9.6 x wt in kg) + (1.8 x ht in cm) – (4.7 x age in years).

Activity Multiplier

Determining our activity multiplier is not black and white like determining our BMR and requires making a judgment call on our part by "rating" our level of daily physical activity. Measurements are broken down into the following categories: sedentary, lightly active, moderately active, very active, and extremely active. Each has its own set value, ranging from 1.2 to 1.9. When this number is multiplied by our BMR, our TCN can be determined. The breakdown of the different categories and their multipliers follows:

1. **Sedentary** = 1.2 (little or no exercise and working a desk job)
2. **Lightly active** = 1.375 (light exercise or sports, one to three days/ week)
3. **Moderately active** = 1.55 (moderate exercise or sports, three to five days/week)
4. **Very active** = 1.725 (hard exercise or sports, six to seven days/ week)
5. **Extremely active** = 1.9 (hard daily exercise or sports *and* physical job or twice-daily training sessions [i.e., marathon, sporting event, etc.])

For example, we will compute the TCN for a woman who is aged thirty, is five foot six, is moderately active, and weighs 120 pounds. To find her TCN, we will need to first find her BMR, derive her activity level, and then multiply the two:

BMR
Women: 655 + (9.6 x wt in kg) + (1.8 x ht in cm) − (4.7 x age in years).
BMR = 655 + 523 + 302 − 141, or 1339 calories daily
Activity level
Moderately active= 1.55
Then, we find our TCN:
TCN: BMR X Activity Multiplier
1139 calories per day x 1.55 = 2,075 total calories needed each day

Absolutely key to determining our calorie intake is to note that BMR and activity level are the principal factors in determining our total calorie needs. We need to keep these in mind as we create our new lifestyle and eating habits. Always remember that if we consume more calories than our TCN, we will gain weight. However, if we eat less than our TCN, we can also harm our health and even gain fat as our body's systems plan to enter "starvation" mode.

A Faster Way to Determine Daily Calorie Intake
If you are in a rush, or just want a "ballpark" idea of your daily calorie needs, there is a faster and easier method to determine your total calorie needs besides using the Harris-Benedict formula above—although it is slightly less accurate than the more involved version.

To quickly determine your total daily calories, calculate twelve to thirteen calories to consume per day for each pound of body weight, *when you are looking to lose fat.* (For a 180-pound person, looking to lose fat, he or she will have to consume approximately 12 x 180, or 2,160 calories per day, when partaking in some moderate physical activity.) However, if you are *seeking to maintain your current weight* and end up within your healthy weight range, consume approximately fifteen to sixteen calories per pound of body weight. (In our example, a 180-pound person who wants to maintain his or her current weight would need to consume approximately 15 x 180, or 2,340 calories per day, when paired with moderate physical activity.) And although it is not as common, if you are looking *for weight gain, consume approximately eighteen to nineteen calories per pound of bodyweight.*

Please note that the Harris-Benedict formula will give you a better approximation of your total calorie needs—and help you reach your goals quicker and more efficiently—but the pared down formula described here is also effective.

The Quality of Our Calories Matter

To create healthy, easy-to-follow habits that last a lifetime, for a diet and lifestyle change, another quick way for determining your daily calorie intake is to decide which type is best for you. Fat loss and maintenance of your current weight are generally the best and healthiest options for people.

Keep in mind that there is much more in food to consider than just calories. For example, there is a difference between eating just calorie-dense food—with few to no nutrients—versus consuming nutrient-rich food. Oftentimes, nutrient-dense foods include significant amounts of vitamins, minerals, and nutrients, while calorie-dense foods often have little nutritional value, if any. Remember that the more foods/beverages you consume that aren't nutrient-rich, the harder it will be for you to obtain the optimal amounts of nutrients without gaining weight. Conversely, vitamins, minerals, nutrients, and water contain zero calories, but are essential for your body to perform its basic functions.

The Importance of Water

Water is not important to our survival—it is essential. In fact, water actually makes up about two-thirds of our body mass. To maintain optimal health, the average adult should drink eight to ten glasses every day. Doing so keeps your body properly hydrated, as well as filling our stomach quite a bit before a meal. We can meet our body's daily water requirement by eating water-rich fruits and vegetables—and to a lesser extent, meats, grains, oats, and rice, other "whole foods," healthy choices, that each have some natural water content. Watery or watery-crisp foods that are high in cholesterol and/or fiber are essential for our good health.

Making wiser food choices, like the ones above, will automatically cut your caloric intake. Again, using the example of a 2,000 calorie per daily intake, we should eat only twenty grams or less of saturated fat (approximately 10 percent or less of your daily calorie intake). However, all fats are not the same. For example, switching from whole to low-fat milk will save you approximately forty-four calories per cup (146 calories to 102 calories). Choosing extra lean ground beef instead of regular will save you eighty-eight calories per three-ounce serving (from 236 calories to 148 calories)—not to mention a reduction of three and a half grams of fat! You can further cut fat yourself by taking the skin from poultry or trimming the fat from any piece of meat.

As we mentioned in our introduction, cooking methods dramatically impact the healthiness of our food. Always try to broil, bake, or roast your meat whenever possible. Frying—as we do with so many of our Desi foods—adds a tremendous amount of oil and grease. For example, baking fish (instead of frying it) will cut out sixty-four calories and 1.3 fat grams in a three-ounce piece. If you enjoy a sizeable piece of cheese (for example, nine ounces of cheddar cheese), changing to low-fat from regular will cut out more than sixty calories, and 4.8 fat grams. In fact, even changing your table spread will make a significant difference: cutting out fat-laden butter and using a trans-fat-free, soft margarine will eliminate nine calories and 1.7 grams of fat (for each tablespoon!), allowing you more calories to use in selecting healthier, tastier foods. Likewise, light salad dressing, low-fat mayonnaise, and vegetable oils are ideal ways to choose healthy without drastically changing your eating choices.

Little Changes Add Up Quickly

The problem with almost every so-called "diet" on the market now is that they fail to recognize the differences that little changes make. Cutting just fifty to one hundred calories per day—and you can see from the examples above that this is not too difficult—is enough to reduce the gradual weight gain that plagues most American and Desi adults.

Furthermore, cutting approximately five hundred calories per day, when carried out properly, can result in weight loss. In fact, cutting your calories by only 15 to 20 percent below your TCN (total calorie need) is a great starting point. (This is only a starting point: this will vary depending upon many factors, as we have already discussed.) However, please note, for most people, cutting your calories by eight hundred or more calories per day will result in the body protecting itself from automatic weight loss. Here, the endocrine glands and your body will tend to purposely slow down your metabolism, restrict your bodily activities, lower your thyroid output, facilitate lean mass loss, and drop the body's initiative to conserve energy when it feels it is becoming calorie-deprived.

Your body has its own reserves of carbohydrates, fat, and protein. How much hunger you have at any given time is impacted by how much you have depleted these reserves. But if you then consume more calories than your body actually requires, the excess can be stored into energy, heat the body, or induce a wide variety of physical activities. And if you consume fewer calories than your body needs to replenish what it used, it will automatically dip into its energy storage to harness unutilized stores, including carbohydrates, fats, or proteins. Doing so creates less heat for the body to make up the difference. Keep in mind that some foods are more easily stored than others, yet an excess of anything is not good. Even healthy foods, when overeaten, are stored as fat. This is alarming, because every pound of fat equals thirty-five thousand calories. However, if you can create your own "calorie deficit" over one week just five hundred calories per day via exercise, diet, or both, you can lose one pound of excess body fat.

The body's reaction to starvation mode is important, because when the body is shorted in any one nutrient or vitamin, the immune system may become weak and have difficulty staving off infections. Additionally, your brain may work slower, and once the body gets to a point where it is undernourished or malnourished, the heart may often begin to pump improperly, deplete its energy stores to perform vital functions, and can even result in death. It is crucial here to note that even though you may consume enough calories, if your food choices are poor, you can still be malnourished or even undernourished. And this is why, whether you are in our modern American culture or a traditional Desi world, there are many, many people who are overweight and still undernourished.

Becoming a Label-Reader

As we mentioned, it is absolutely essential that you become a label-reader when it comes to your food and beverage consumption. Thankfully, America is much more stringent about their food labeling guidelines than Desi lands. Here, food and beverage manufacturers must label their products with calorie guides. Yes, there are some loopholes (the ability to label anything between ½ gram to 0 grams per serving of trans-fat as "0 g trans-fat" comes to mind). Similarly, the "Daily Value" information label is based on a 2,000-calorie per day diet, which is just a rough estimate and not the same for each and every person. Labels are useful in that they show serving size, calories, calories from fat, nutrients that need to be limited, and nutrients that require increased levels, as well as a detailed footnote illustrating the daily value percent of each nutrient present in the food (and listed on the label). In general, nutrients that we should limit are: trans and saturated fat, cholesterol, and sodium. Nutrients that are essential and hence, need to be increased are fiber, vitamins A & C, calcium, iron, as well as other vitamins and minerals.

These daily food requirements are set by our Food and Drug Administration (or FDA). However, the FDA's idea of a serving size is pretty small by today's standards. You would be well off to observe your actual portions for a few days to see if they match the suggested serving sizes found on your foods' labels. Note that when your portion is smaller or larger than the label's serving amount, the food's value will change and can give you an excess or shortage of calories. This is important, because according to the FDA's guide to daily value percentages, 5 percent or less of a given food is considered a "low source" of that nutrient; 20 percent or more is considered too high. Being wary of these suggestions, guides, and labels will help you make better-informed decisions *before* you pack on inches around your waistline. Not surprisingly, restaurants are trying to keep pace or in some areas, like New York City, being forced into placing some kind of calorie guide posted on their menus to inform their patrons of their prepared foods' calorie content.

Enacting What You Have Learned

So you're ready to start cutting calories and get out there and start walking a half-hour per day. Let's get started, right? *Not so fast.* Before changing your diet or beginning an exercise regimen, contact your physician to see if your body can handle these changes. If your doctor okays it, be sure to discuss with him or her the specifics of such a plan. Determining your proper activity level should always involve your medical professional, particularly when you have been living a sedentary lifestyle for years (or decades)!

Once you have your doctor's permission and are ready to go, be sure to first note both your body weight and body fat percentage. Knowing these will allow you to figure out precisely how you are responding to your new plan. As we will discuss in detail later on, a food and exercise journal will allow you to keep track of your daily calorie consumption, how many servings of suggested food groups you consume, the physical activities you partake in, and your mood and mental well-being. By paying close attention to your activities and their intensity and length, you will have a clearer picture of the calories you burn each week. Additionally, this journal has practical benefits. It is the perfect place in which to jot down ideas for meals and recipes, as well as your schedule. Following your progress will give you pride and bolster your confidence as you see, in black and white, the progress you have made.

Keeping a journal will also help you quickly identify the reason behind any time you get sidetracked. There may be times when you need to decrease your calorie consumption or increase your physical activity depending upon how your body reacts to your new plan. Always keep in mind that gradual weight loss and muscle gain are optimal. Quick weight loss and the regimens that facilitate them are not recommended because they are often unhealthy, and they often promote "yo-yo" reactions, at the least. Once your steady nutrition and exercise plan are established, you may best determine how to set and maintain a negative calorie balance.

A negative calorie balance occurs when you are burning off more calories than you are taking in.

Maintaining a negative calorie balance is a vital part of the *Desi Diet*. In the long run, calories coming in must be less than calories being used for the body's energy to enable sustained weight loss.

The Importance of Exercise

We will mention this many times throughout the *Desi Diet*, because it is so true: the importance of regular physical activity, even walking or chores, cannot be overestimated. I was reminded of this fact on a recent trip back to my roots in Pakistan.

While visiting my uncle in Lahore, I was assigned a driver who would drive me around wherever I wanted to go. This guy was a pretty massive person. He definitely had some fat on him, but you could also tell that under the fat was some serious solid muscle. I was inspired to see the countryside of Lahore, so I called him up and told him that tomorrow morning we would hit the countryside and pick up some breakfast on the way. Just before the sun came up, he was at my door. I got into the car, and off we went. Our first stop was to this little shop on the side of the street where we picked up some lassi and parata. The lassi was so thick you could almost eat it with a spoon. I barely could finish my cup of lassi and parata. However, the driver downed two cups of lassi and several paratas as if they were just a warm-up.

While we were finishing up breakfast, some girls came running over who apparently knew the driver, asking for some help .We walked over through some fields to find that there was a water buffalo stuck in the mud. The driver proceeded to walk into the mud and lift the water buffalo out of the mud. It was probably the most impressive show of strength I have ever seen! After the water buffalo was out of the mud, we went back to truck and headed off to the hills. Once we got to the location, we started our hike. Within a few hours, I could start to feel fatigue from climbing so many hills. Even with my hiking boots and all the latest gear, I was having a tough time making it up the hills. The driver, on the other hand, was wearing slippers and no gear at all—and was having no trouble at all. Later, I found out that he was born in a little village in the hills. Eventually we got to the village where he was born. Here, I noticed that everyone was pretty muscular. And although their diets were loaded with fat and carbohydrates, they still maintained pretty good physical structures. I realized then that everything they did involved burning lots of calories.

Most of the townspeople did not own cars, so they walked everywhere; to get to the nearest store, you had to walk halfway up a large hill. And even when they wanted to sell goods they produced in the village, they would drag a homemade, wooden-wheeled wagon several miles into the nearest town, walking around all day to sell their wares. But with such a physically demanding lifestyle, they had developed great muscular structures regardless of what they ate. I submit that story to you so that you may always remember that diet is only ever half the equation of a healthy lifestyle change.

Moving Forward

Beginning a healthy lifestyle today will help you, your loved ones, and your family both now and in the future. Obesity has been proven to cause diseases, illnesses, and other health problems. Stroke, type-2 diabetes, heart disease, heart attacks, and premature death are just a few of the many health problems that can be prevented by enacting a healthy lifestyle. When this lifestyle includes eating the proper foods, sticking to your optimal calorie intake, and maintaining regular physical activity, you will maintain a healthy weight range. And regardless of whether you lose, maintain, or gain weight, your primary concern should be your physical and mental health, not only your physical appearance. By making the decision to commit to a healthy lifestyle change, you are going a long way toward breaking the cycle of weight issues and constant flux.

Remember that by following the Desi Diet, you are embarking on a lifestyle change—not a short-term fad or adjustment. To maintain a healthy weight range, it is important to balance your food and beverage calories you take in during the day with the amount of calories your body expends. This balance is a critical portion of the ratio between calories consumed and calories used by the body throughout the day for energy. For example, if you consume a food with 300 calories and your body only uses 150 calories for digestion, its basal metabolic rate will be an excess of 150 calories stored in your energy reserves—and that will more than likely be stored as body fat. Counting calories is an important aspect of making this healthy lifestyle change because it helps with weight and fat loss. When paired with a proper nutritional plan and exercise regime, the results can be profound.

Remember that the number of calories you consume directly affects your metabolism. Thus it is important not to load your calorie count with "empty" calories to keep up a higher metabolism. Assessing your food's nutritional value as well as calories is essential. Cutting nutrient-dense foods, no matter how many calories they may have, is never as important as cutting out the "empty" calories lacking nutritional value. Wiser food choices will allow you to still enjoy foods you love—and cut calories and fats via portion control. Choosing nutritious foods and keeping the portion sizes under control are powerful weapons in the battle against the bulge.

Remember that the technical definition of a calorie is the quantity of heat required to raise the temperature of 1 gram of water just 1 degree Celsius from a standard initial temperature. But as it applies to nutrition—and for the purposes of the Desi Diet—a calorie is defined as a unit of energy-producing potential equal to this quantity of heat that is contained in food and released upon oxidation by the body. A calorie is the standard measure of nutrition and critical when considering your health and food consumption. The calorie is the building block of our energy consumption, overall health—and its properties set the foundation for much of the *Desi Diet.*

Tapering Meal Size

True, Americans are finally catching onto the importance of eating better. Yet still, the average American town or city creates a toxic landscape that makes it hard for us to stay healthy. Everywhere you turn are drive-through fast-food restaurants; convenience stores open 24/7 with their sixty-four-ounce jumbo sodas; and "family" restaurants that provide gigantic-sized portions, roughly twice what a typical portion size was just a few decades ago. And our modern on-the-go lifestyle doesn't help any either; we're more likely to eat at an airport, in the car, in front of the TV, or at our desk at work than we are to sit down for a leisurely family dinner. This fixation with large portions is also, in part, driven by our need as a culture to skip breakfast.

As Desis, we are pretty similar to our American counterparts. I am from the city of Karachi in Pakistan. I grew up in the States, but when I go back to visit, I have found that in general and particularly when people don't have to go to work, they sleep pretty late. It is common to just skip breakfast and have some chai (tea) once they wake up. However, as we discussed earlier, this immediately sends the body into a state of shock, slowing down our metabolic rate. A normal day back home may consist of visiting friends and family for chai and crackers. But if you're Desi, you know that (more often than not) crackers are replaced by some random fried food. Since our culture is very big on being a good host, it is mandatory to feed our guests—and it is just as important for that guest to eat or he or she will be considered rude. And unfortunately, the most important meal of the day ends up being dinner where every family member (and our ever-present guests) will get together and sit and eat (and eat some more).

Lahore is another very popular city of Pakistan that is known for its food. Many nights they even close down the streets and have vendors selling food all night long; one particularly famous street is called simply, "Food Street." Step inside a restaurant around 8:00 or 9:00 p.m. and you'll find it empty; step onto the streets at midnight and you'll find thousands of people eating all sorts of (mostly fried) treats. The norm here, and throughout the subcontinent, is to eat late in the evening and then pretty much go right to bed. However, despite this, I have found that people in Pakistan and India tend to be thinner in appearance compared to the Desi population here in the United States. Perhaps that's because one thing they don't have in the South Asian countries is the extensive amount of hormones and preservatives commonly found in American food. Likewise, combining the lifestyle of back home and mixing it with the hormones and preservatives of the food here has been expanding our collective waistline.

The Importance of Breakfast to a Healthy Lifestyle

"Eat breakfast like a king, lunch like a prince, and dinner like a pauper."
— old German proverb

Okay, so I'm Desi, but I'll take my proverbs (and wisdom) where I can get them. Think of it like this: breakfast means *breaking* the *fast*. By eating breakfast, we immediately bring our blood sugar levels back to normal and jumpstart our metabolism. Conversely, those of us who skip breakfast on a regular basis tend to eat more throughout the day, eat larger dinners (*sound like you and your Desi friends described above?*), and go on carb-driven eating binges. Perhaps worst of all, skipping breakfast causes us to eat more before going to bed, which in turn causes us to pack on the pounds, as our metabolism is resting and can't digest this food.

In short, we cannot overstate the importance of eating breakfast. But this doesn't mean stuffing ourselves with anything in the fridge. Good common sense and moderation applies here, as with all nutritional issues. Additionally, there is one key caveat to this rule: eat breakfast within one hour of waking. This will help to set the body's natural metabolic functioning on its natural pace and prevent those cravings later in the day. In fact, multiple studies have found that people who skip breakfast tend to eat more food overall, have higher cholesterol levels, and become more insulin-resistant—which are all precursors to weight gain, heart disease, and diabetes.

Leverage the Power of Breakfast to Keep Your Metabolism Going

Once you begin eating breakfast regularly and within an hour of waking, you'll automatically begin to feel your energy levels increase. Leverage this newly tapped power by expanding upon it throughout the day. Try the following tips:

- Instead of eating three large meals per day, eat six smaller ones
- Eat every three hours, alternating between meals and snacks
- Stop eating three hours before bedtime.

Eating six times per day, approximately three hours apart, will help to keep your metabolism running smoothly throughout the day, which will gradually reduce cravings for sweets and other carb-laden foods. Additionally, if you can stop eating three hours before you go to sleep, you are giving your body the time it needs to digest the food before bedtime. That way the food is used to power your normal body functions instead of immediately going to sleep, when the food is digested in your sleep and stored as fat.

Another Common Eating Rule Shattered (Sort of . . .)

Just as we have shown that eating a decent breakfast, contrary to popular belief and/or common practice, is actually healthy, there is another common rule about eating that is widely misunderstood. Sure, we know that (from our chapter on calories) losing weight is based on burning more calories than we take in. There is an equally important addition to this rule that is always often ignored with typical "diets."

Although we must burn more calories than we take in to lose weight, if we eat too few calories, we will actually not lose weight, because we fail to turn on our body's metabolism.

We talked earlier about how our bodies since the beginning of our history and continuing through to today are hardwired to go into starvation mode when we don't eat enough calories. (From our prehistoric forbearers, the body thinks that we are preparing for a long period without food, and the body automatically lowers its metabolism and stores up on fat.) The World Health Organization classifies a starvation diet as anything less than 2,100 calories per day for the average male and 1,800 calories per day for the average female.[3] Then consider this: the average American on a diet is eating somewhere between 1,500 and 1,800 calories per day.

So what are we doing when we diet? We restrict our caloric intake, which sets our body into starvation mode, burning muscle and holding on for dear life to its fat. Since we're not eating enough, we are in a constant state of nervousness, are tempted to overeat, eat the wrong foods, and eat late at night. Welcome to the definition of yo-yo diet, which is exactly why, despite its name, the *Desi Diet* is a lifestyle change and not a diet.

Most of us are educated enough to know that eating, say, four thousand calories a day will cause us to gain weight. But contrary to popular belief, eating too little, even as much as fifteen hundred calories a day, will wreak as much havoc on our bodies. The key is to eat slightly *above* what is called our resting metabolic rate, forcing our body to continually have our metabolism turned on, being the natural, calorie-burning engine that it can be.

Resting Metabolic Rate is the basic amount of energy (i.e., calories) that it takes to run your body's metabolism for one day. A good rule of thumb for the average person is your Resting Metabolic Rate (RMR) is about *ten times* your weight in pounds. For example, I weigh 150 pounds, so my RMR is 1,500 calories, which means I should eat approximately eleven times my weight in calories to maximize my body's fat-burning powers (or 11 x 150 = 1,650 calories).

If Dr. Noor were to eat less than 1,650 calories per day, his body would go into starvation mode, and he would begin burning muscle, hanging onto fat, and in general, feeling a loss of energy. However, if he ups this to 1,650 calories per day, he will naturally lose fat, have more energy, and keep more muscle mass (which is exactly what he has done, and why he continues to remain in good health).

Some Powerful Eating Tips

So far in this chapter, we have discussed the importance of eating breakfast within one hour of waking, eating six smaller meals throughout the day, and stopping eating at least three hours before going to bed at night. The following tips will also help you:

- **Take control of your hunger:** When you feel hunger pangs, try to stop and ask yourself, *am I really hungry?* If you're not really sure, wait twenty minutes and ask yourself again. Most times you'll find that, by simply being aware of your cravings, you can take control of them.

- **Use the power of snacks:** Many times you will find that a small snack will be enough to tide you over until your next meal. If you are having trouble with food cravings, make sure to have ready-to-eat fruits, vegetables, nuts, or other simple snacks on hand. A healthy snack will serve to satisfy your hunger and kick start your metabolism as well.

- **Institute a "stop" control:** It's no secret that many of us in our on-the-go, 24/7 world eat simultaneously while performing another activity. The problem here is that, in these times, we have no "stop signal" that tells us when it is time to stop eating. If our mind is focused on another activity—be that watching the tube, surfing the web, or chatting with a friend on the phone—we can be tricked and keep eating, even though we are full.

- **Sit down and eat (and only eat):** Building on the point above, unless you are eating in the company of others, sit down at the table to eat. That's it. No computer, no phone calls, etc. Doing this will not only allow you to actually enjoy your food, but you will also tend to pay better attention to your hunger signals.

- **Get out of the "low-fat zone":** Think low-fat means fewer calories? Wrong. Oftentimes, the exact opposite is true. Check your food labels. Most often low-fat foods—to mask the blandness that comes when fat is removed—are actually high in sugar and are still high in calories.

- **Ditch the giant dishes (and the wide glasses):** Unfortunately, we Desis and Americans have a tendency to put whatever food is in front of us into our mouths. If you happen to serve your food in an extra-large bowl, plate, or dish, you are just increasing the odds that you will overeat. Try smaller-sized dishes for a few weeks, and see if you notice any differences around your waistline. And consider this: multiple studies prove that when people pour juice into two shapes of glasses (short and wide vs. tall and thin), they will fill the short one to the top and only fill the tall one halfway. Since the glasses still hold the same amount, choosing the short one will mean you consume more juice than if you had chosen the tall one (which is only halfway full). So the next time you reach for a glass, go for a taller, thinner one. You may actually save yourself fifty to one hundred calories or so.

- **Keep Treats Out Of Sight:** Even the most-disciplined of us with no health or food issues at all may be tempted to eat when food is in front of us "just because." So take charge of your surroundings. If you're going to leave food out around your home, make sure that it's healthy food, at least. That way, if you're tempted to eat, you'll find yourself digging into a bowl of fruit as opposed to a bag of chips.

Consciously Make Food a Part of Your Lifestyle

When you're enjoying that second helping of *bagaara baingan, dumm aloo, tanddor chickeni*—or just plain old burger, fries, or pizza—ask yourself, *is this really worth it?* Try visualizing the consequences of eating too much. Do you really want to spend an extra hour at the gym to work off those calories that come with that second helping? Are you happy to add a half-inch around your waist because you have a big project this week and are skipping breakfast all week and overeating at dinnertime?

It is quite unnerving, honestly, how much work can be involved to burn off the food that we can consume in just one sitting. If you can internalize this fact, you may suddenly find that food is not quite as enjoyable; if so, you will turn down that second helping. You will do so knowing that the instant gratification that comes along with tasting, smelling, and eating food doesn't beat out the toll it will exact on your health. Remembering this concept can be the best way to create an automatic, ingrained aversion to overeating.

The Social Aspects of Food

We don't have to remind you of the afternoon chai with friends that stretches into a day of socializing and overeating. Yes, as Desis, food is inextricably interwoven with our culture, but there's no reason we can't use this in social settings to actually help us in our healthy lifestyle. When you were younger, it might have been your mother who pushed that extra serving of *naan*, but now that you're an adult, you can use your social relationships in your favor. When Mom comes to visit these days, don't be afraid to ask her to stop bringing sweets, as an example.

Eating in the workplace has its own particular set of hazards, as well. Have you ever gone along with what everyone is doing just to be part of the fun, whether that means going for pizza and soda or having a slice of cake at the umpteenth coworker birthday celebration? Remember that you *do* have a choice. Even if you decide to join your work buddies at the fast-food restaurant, you can order a salad or yogurt. Or you can be even more assertive and suggest a healthier venue altogether. Of course, if you've worked in any type of job long enough, you'll be faced with the inevitable all-you-can-eat buffet. Instead of piling your plate high with a little bit of everything and fried, fat-laden foods, pick one healthy dish and actually enjoy yourself.

You may already know that, for many people, food and health have their own set of issues as well. When dealing with family, your spouse or partner may feel that exercise cuts down on your time together or even feel threatened by your sudden new interest in maintaining a healthy lifestyle. In those instances, instead of fighting with him or her, suggest that the two of you take a walk together, and then relax in front of the tube or better yet, come home and prepare a healthy meal together.

Visiting with friends and relatives, particularly during the holidays, can be a complete assault on any healthy eating patterns you've established and truly test your resolve. Again, use that social connection to strengthen your healthy lifestyle, not hurt it. Offer to bring a dish for everyone to share. Not only is that the considerate thing to do, but you'll also guarantee that you have at least one healthy eating option available. And if you know sugar-laden sodas are in the plans, set a limit ahead of time, and then be prepared to make the switch to water or juice instead.

Last, do your best not to make socializing just about the food. Enjoy your food, eat healthy, but don't be afraid to move on and celebrate the social aspects of any event. Be assertive and move the focus off food. Go out dancing, play a sport together, or just go for a walk. Think of creative ways to transform your current social patterns into activities that have a more positive impact on your health and well being.

Why You Need to Set Goals

You probably already use goal-setting in your personal and professional life. And although we realize the value of goal-setting, many of us, when it comes to weight loss and our overall health, are stuck—due precisely to poor goal-setting. Taking the time to actually set goals now will dramatically increase your chances of achieving long-term healthiness. Below are five important things to remember:

1. **Work in small steps:** It can become demoralizing quickly when you set lofty goals and then fail to achieve them. If you say you want to lose sixty pounds, you may become daunted by the sheer amount of effort you perceive that taking and lose your will, or even put on weight out of frustration. However, losing five pounds a month for the next ten months may be a practical (and, in fact, inspiring) goal to achieve.

2. **Be specific:** Take time to ask yourself the right questions, and get as specific as possible: Do you want to lose weight or just body fat? How much, and more importantly, why? Do you want to change the foods you are eating? If so, what foods will you be replacing them with? Do you have recipes and meals that you'll actually want to eat, that will keep you inspired? When you ask yourself pointed, focused questions, you stand a better chance of reaching your goals.

3. **Be realistic:** Do you have the time to put into a six-day a week workout routine? If not, a more realistic but steady three or four days per week are better than none. Are you obsessed with losing every last inch of body fat? Then take time to remember the lightest weight you ever were in your life. Although our TV commercials and magazine ads may try to prove otherwise, there are actually different body types. Not every woman will fit into a size-zero dress or every man into a thirty-two-inch pair of jeans. If you weren't those dimensions when you were eighteen, it's unrealistic to think that you can obtain that size now, in your twenties, thirties, forties, or beyond.

4. **Focus within:** I have said it many times: the *Desi Diet* is much more than a diet; it's a lifestyle change. Likewise, when you set goals, try to shift the focus toward things you can change, like your attitude, mindset, and lifestyle goals. Don't dwell on the past or on your starting point. Create positive thoughts on where you're going and how much fun and joy it will bring for you to

get there. This is absolutely critical to long-term success. If you haven't begun to do so already, use guided imagery on a daily basis. Create a few positive thoughts where you envision yourself eating healthfully, exercising regularly, and feeling better about yourself. Use these, and repeat them early in the day and often throughout the day.

5. **Realize it now—there will be setbacks:** Remember that there is never any perfectly seamless journey in life. The key point is to create an action plan that keeps you balanced, motivated, and on track. Map out sections that may distract you from your exercise routine or eating plan and create solutions, now, before you have to act. This will enable you to be prepared being prepared for jumping back on your game quickly, figuring out why and how the setback occurred, and what you can learn from the experience.

The Importance of "Cheat Days"

We keep repeating how the *Desi Diet* is in fact a lifestyle change and not a diet. While even a lifestyle change is beneficial, it may be difficult for even the most disciplined of us, to "forget" everything from our old lifestyle. One great way to keep some remnant of your old self around is to have a "cheat day." In essence, it's a day where you can eat whatever you want and not follow any particular schedule. You may choose to do this as intensely as you desire, from eating anything in sight to just having a special dessert after a healthy meal.

The cheat day has two main benefits:

o In the beginning, and until you reach your desired body composition, a cheat day will help you adjust physically, and perhaps more importantly, mentally, to the new lifestyle.

o A cheat day will actually serve to *reset* your metabolism, considering the fact that the human body is always trying (naturally, on its own) to adapt to change.

In general, the leaner you become, the more cheat meals or days might be needed to get to this "revved up" point. However, to ensure that you don't end up just eating tremendous amounts of junk food, you might want to eat more carbohydrates, one of the body's main sources of fuel. When you are considering how much and when to cheat, you should also take the time to look at how this cheating will affect your psyche. Some people feel that cheating allows them to positively deal with the shift to a new lifestyle. However, there can be negative effects, as well. Some people use their cheat day as an excuse to "pig out" so extremely that they are putting themselves at an increased health risk; others, who start actually fantasizing about the cheat day days ahead of time, may be at increased risk for developing an eating disorder. In either case, you should stop and call your physician.

For those beginning their cheat day, I would suggest the following:

- Start with a cheat day once a week
- After one month, switch to having a cheat day once every two weeks
- Finally, try just one cheat meal once every two weeks.

In my own personal life, if I am getting ready for a martial arts competition and I have to make a certain weight class, I will have a cheat meal every fourteen days, which throws my metabolism into overdrive. I have found the impact of instituting cheat days to be incredibly powerful. Since I no longer eat fast foods and my cheat meals are just large servings of pasta, I have found myself actually disliking the smell of French fries and other fried food.

The Importance of Dinner

Although we have mentioned it before, the idea cannot be stressed enough: as a society, we are killing ourselves by making dinner the main meal of our day. Eating (mostly) unhealthy, processed foods just hours before sleeping and going to bed almost immediately after dinner just ensures that the food we eat will be stored as fat. And after years and decades of repeating this pattern, we are hurtling ever-faster toward all the diseases plaguing our society, like heart disease, diabetes, cancer, and many others.

Building on other ideas mentioned in this chapter, we can use dinner to reinforce healthy eating patterns with our families. Sitting down to a well-prepared, healthy smaller dinner with friends or family will galvanize your new lifestyle. Being more structured with your meals will not only help you keep in mind how much you are eating (thus tapering their size) but will naturally make you feel better—and as a result, make healthier eating choices, as well.

Food Journals (and Why You Should Be Keeping One)

Keeping a food journal can be one of the most critical things you implement to ensure weight loss success and overall better health. First and foremost, keeping a journal of your daily food intake will create a conscious awareness of your eating patterns, both good and bad. For example, after keeping a daily journal, many people are often surprised to find out what they thought was an "occasional" midnight snack is a three-time-per-week event occurring like clockwork. Remember that there are many things in our lives that are outside of our control; however, we *can* and *do* make choices about what we eat.

For starters, include the following:

- What you eat and drink
- How much you eat or drink, including size, volume, weight, and/or number
- When you eat/drink
- Where you eat/drink
- With whom you eat/drink (or if alone)
- Does your eating include any activities? (Using the computer, watching TV, etc.)
- Your frame of mind: how are you feeling? (Before, during, and after eating)

How to interpret your food journal: After a period of time (a week will usually suffice), take a look at your records. Focus on what your biggest motivations/problem areas are. If your problem is portion-control, examine how much you ate. If you are having problems eating vitamin-rich, nutritious foods, see when and if you are eating those items. If you're not eating enough of them, how come? No matter what your particular issue is, the problem is like every other problem: simply becoming aware of the issue is a significant first step.

You May Be Very Surprised about What You Learn from Your Food Journal

Personally, I discovered some interesting things about myself after keeping a food journal for only a few weeks. Back home, I had been accustomed to sitting down, talking, and relaxing while eating. But here, at least in New York, everything is on the go. Last year, I would pick up a coworker and we'd stop at a deli to get something to eat and drive to work while eating. It wasn't anything I paid attention to at the time, but once I started keeping a journal, I realized what poor decisions I was making at that deli: eating larger portions than normal, eating fatty, salty foods, and consuming too much coffee. Reading back my journal, I realized that I had come to associate stopping at the deli with hunger and the urge to eat. But simply noticing the habit in my journal wasn't enough: to change that habit, I stopped eating in my car. By eating at my desk at work or having breakfast before I leave home, I no longer feel the urge to eat while I drive. And just by sitting down and taking my time while I eat, I find I enjoy my food more and feel fuller for a longer time.

There are discoveries for you regarding your own eating habits; that much I can guarantee you. Don't put off this valuable learning experience for another time. Start your own food journal today.

Water Intake

A few years ago, I was out west, hiking in the northern part of the Mojave Desert in the Death Valley National Park. I was pretty excited, as it was my first time hiking in a desert. Prior to the hiking trip, I had packed my gear: a hydro-backpack with two liters of water, several energy and protein bars, a snake hook, a compass, and fifteen feet of rope. I had only planned on hiking for one day, approximately eight to ten hours. At 6:00 a.m., we started our hike, watching the sun rise as we began. Within two hours, the sun was out in full effect. Since everyone in my group was an avid hiker, we kept a pretty good pace. I couldn't help but noticing that the temperature had risen very quickly. At the halfway point, around noon, we took a short lunch break, where I noticed I had finished all my water. We started to loop back—but within an hour, my legs started to really cramp up. I started to slow down, and within two hours, I was beginning to feel lightheaded. I grabbed an energy bar, but I could barely swallow it; my body was no longer producing saliva or sweat. Finally, we made it back to our truck around 6:00 p.m. What was supposed to be a pleasant if somewhat strenuous day turned into a twelve-hour ordeal. For me, a lifelong fitness buff, I hadn't realized the true value of water until I ran out of it.

Your body needs constant, ongoing water replenishment. Your body consists of 55 percent to 75 percent water; if you have a lean body type, you will have more water, as muscle holds more water than fat. Your body uses up and expels an incredible amount of water each day. Your lungs expel two to four cups of water per day (just through normal breathing!) and even more on colder days. Even your feet sweating is good for another cup of water loss; a half-dozen trips to the bathroom means six cups of water lost. Perspiring, not even including exercise-driven perspiration, will eliminate two cups from your body.

Although the technical definition of dehydration is to lose 10 percent of your body weight in fluids, even as little as 2 percent can hurt your athletic abilities, increase fatigue, and lead to poor memory. Additionally, proper water consumption lessens your chances of developing kidney stones, lubricates joints, prevents/weakens the common cold and flu, and prevents constipation. Symptoms of dehydration, even mild dehydration, can cause the following:

- Increased, excessive thirst
- Fatigue, tiredness
- Headaches
- Dry mouth
- Reduced (or no) urination
- Muscle weakness or pain
- Dizziness or lightheadedness

If you are a healthy man or woman and not subject to any dehydrating conditions, you can usually utilize your thirst to indicate when to drink water. *However, thirst is not always a precise gauge of your body's need for fluids.* In fact, the older you are, the less you will be able to sense that you are thirsty. During vigorous exercise, regardless of your age, a significant amount of your reserve fluids may be depleted before you even feel thirsty. Thus, it is important to thoroughly hydrate yourself before, during, and after physical exertion.

It is important that you pay attention to your body's signals, including thirst. Pronounced thirst and/or increased urination (in frequency or volume) can be early warning signs of diabetes. Here, excess blood sugar, or glucose, draws water from your body's tissues, making you feel dehydrated. And to quench that thirst, you will naturally drink additional water, leading to more frequent urination. *Thus, it is absolutely essential that if you experience unexplained increases in your thirst and urination, you see your doctor.* Thankfully, this may not mean that you have diabetes; some people just naturally consume larger amounts of water and experience increased urine output, not due to any underlying disease.

Healthy Drinking

Above all else, be sure to keep yourself hydrated and select water to drink as much as possible. As always, check with your doctor, but most healthy adults should stick to the following:

- Drink one glass of water with each meal and one between each meal.
- Choose water instead of tea or coffee, as much as possible.
- At social events, pick sparkling water instead of sodas.

If you choose to drink your water from a bottle, be sure to clean and/or replace it often, because when you drink, old contaminants may contaminate the bottle's refilled water. Of course, for our environment's sake, if you use a bottle often, be sure it is a reusable bottle and to clean it, wash it in hot, soapy water.

And although this is rare, it is possible to drink too much water. Doing so can overwhelm your kidneys' natural abilities to eliminate water. This condition eventually leads to hyponatremia, where excess water intake dilutes your blood's normal sodium level. The elderly, people with certain medical conditions (e.g., congestive heart failure and cirrhosis), or who take certain diuretics are at increased risk of hyponatremia.

Drink Water and Lose Weight?

The answer is a resounding *yes!* All of your body's functions require water's presence, so a well-hydrated body only improves the effectiveness of these functions. These millions of processes each involve metabolism; drinking sufficient water boosts your metabolism and improves your energy. In fact, drinking water makes your overall metabolism burn calories 3 percent faster.

Actually, your body has innumerable types of metabolism operating at all times. One critical version is the metabolism of fat, a task completed by the liver when it converts stored fat to energy. (Although the liver has other functions, this is one that is extremely important.) However, another one of its tasks is to fill in for your kidneys. Your kidneys must be properly hydrated to function properly. When the kidneys are water-deprived, your liver has to pick up the slack, thus becoming less productive in its own tasks. It then cannot metabolize fat as fast or effectively when the kidneys were working; when you let this happen, you are burdening your liver—and facilitating the increased amount of fat storage.

Besides the demonstrated boost to metabolism, several studies show your hunger and thirst sensations are triggered simultaneously. Thus, if your body feels even slight dehydration, your perception may mistake this thirst for hunger and trigger you to eat when you truly are not hungry. However, just about every food contains at least some water. When you don't drink, you may be pushed to eat more and gain the needed water supply (not to mention the additional calories). Simply put: when you drink the proper amount of water, your body will less likely be "tricked" into thinking it is hungry. As a result, you will eat less and lose weight.

This link between hunger and thirst are particularly important given today's typical modern diet. Many foods created today contain incredible amounts of added sugars, extra fats, and insufficient water. A major cause is that, today, foods are typically stored for a long period of time. Therefore, we eat less of foods with high water content like milk, fruits, or yogurt, for example, because they spoil quickly. The truth is that many popular fad diets today do not calculate enough water consumption, and because of the amounts of processed, fried, and hydrogenated food, it is more important than ever that we drink more water to reduce our food cravings.

How Much Water Is Enough?

There is no tried and true amount of water that each of us should drink each day. That is because although water is critical to our health, our precise needs vary from person to person. There is no one decisive study on the matter; our daily water recommendation is in fact based on your overall health, activity levels, and where you live. Since there is no exact formula, it is all the more important that you learn more about the matter. Every day your breath, perspiration, urine, and bowel movements account for substantial water loss. However, for your body to run at its peak performance level, you must continually replenish this water supply by drinking water and consuming foods and drinks that also contain water. The following methods approximate the daily water requirements for the average, healthy adult.

The replacement approach: Typical adults average 1.5 liters (6.3 cups) of urine output daily. You also lose approximately an additional liter of water via bowel movements, breathing, and sweating. Since food typically accounts for 20 percent of total fluid intake, if you consume two liters of beverages per day (a bit over eight cups) along with your food, you will replace the lost fluids.

Eight eight-ounce glasses of water daily: The "eight x eight rule," or drinking eight eight-ounce glasses of water (or 1.9 liters) daily is a good rule of thumb, as well. Although this rule is not supported by as much scientific evidence as the one above, it is still a valid basic guideline that many people practice with beneficial results.

Dietary-focused: Many studies recommend that men consume three liters (about thirteen cups) and women consume 2.2 liters (about nine cups) of total beverages daily.

Besides these three guidelines, if you drink enough fluid that you do not feel thirsty very much, and produce approximately 1.5 liters (6.3 cups) or more of colorless or slightly yellow urine daily, your water intake is most likely sufficient.

Factors Influencing Your Water Needs

As we mentioned, there are three main factors affecting your total daily water intake requirements.

Exercise: When you exercise or partake in physical activity that causes you to sweat, you must drink extra water to make up for the resultant fluid loss. For shorter exercise periods, an additional one and a half to two and a half cups of water is sufficient. For longer, intense exercise lasting sixty minutes or more (competing in a marathon, as an example), you must drink more than this. And this additional amount will be affected by how much sweat you produce, the length of exercise, and the type of physical activity. Drinking juice is a poor option, because juices tend to have excess sugars and chemicals. A sports drink will ensure that you replace the sweat and slash the risk of developing hyponatremia, a life-threatening condition. It is also important to continue to replace fluids after your exercise is over.

Environment: Additional water is also required when you are out in humid or hot climates, causing sweat. (Heated indoor air may have the same effect.) Additionally, extreme altitudes (8,200 feet of higher) can set off increased urination and rapid breathing, which tend to deplete critical water reserves.

Illnesses and other health conditions: Illness symptoms, like fever, vomiting, or diarrhea, cause your body to lose additional fluids. Here, you should increase water consumption—and in extreme cases, consider a re-hydration solution, like CeraLyte. Some conditions, such as urinary tract infections or kidney stones, may demand an increased water intake. Conversely, conditions like heart failure and some kidney, liver, and adrenal diseases may hinder water excretion and even dictate decreased water intake.

Pregnancy and breastfeeding: Expectant women or those who are breastfeeding require additional water to remain hydrated; your body uses very large amounts of fluid, particularly when nursing. The current recommendation is that expecting women should consume approximately ten cups of fluids daily; those breastfeeding should consume about thirteen cups of fluids daily.

Additional Water Sources

While you might try to keep a water bottle within reach 24/7, that is just not practical. Additionally, you just don't need to. Your foods provide a considerable portion of your daily water needs, particularly if you are eating plenty of healthy fruits and leafy green vegetables. In fact, even a reasonably healthy diet provides approximately 20 percent of your total water intake (the balance comes from water and all sorts of beverages).

The importance of healthy fruits and vegetables cannot be overstated: tomatoes and watermelons, for example, are more than 90 percent water, by weight. Regarding beverages, coffee, tea, and soda do have water, but they should not be counted on, because they often have caffeine, sugars, and even unhealthy chemicals.

Implementing Your Proper Water Intake Amount

Be prepared. You will probably find yourself running to the bathroom constantly in the first few days of drinking more water than usual. Perhaps you will even feel annoyed or frustrated. But have patience: your body is now flushing out all the excess water it has stored over all those years (or decades) of living in "starvation mode." You may not realize it, but your body is undergoing a radical transformation. As you give your body all the water it needs, it will eliminate that which is unneeded. It may flush out all of that excess water surrounding your hips, ankles, and yes, even your gut. Your body is in fact realizing that it no longer has to save these stores. It instinctively, unfailingly trusts that the water will continue to come. And eventually, your body's flushing will cease (and your life will return to normal).

Remember that only water has the powerful flushing effect. In fact, even though one recent study showed that caffeine increases your body's fat-burning potential over the long run, the opposite is true. Caffeine is, in fact, a diuretic that causes your body to dehydrate. While caffeine *will* increase heart rate (and in the process, burn some additional calories), this actually ends up hurting you—because your muscles need water to function properly. And the combination of caffeine and physical activity isn't particularly good for your heart; your heart is already working hard enough.

Finding the Right Water Temperature

Both cold and warm water have their benefits. Cold water is absorbed by the stomach more quickly, and some studies have shown that it assists your body's fat-burning abilities. However, warm water is easier to drink in large amounts. But the key point to remember is that regardless of temperature, drinking water is critical.

Water: Nature's Beauty Secret

The old wives' tale that water will help improve your looks is actually true. Water flushes out your skin's impurities, resulting in a glowing, clearer complexion. Additionally, saggy skin (caused by weight-loss or age) fills out nicely when its cells become properly hydrated. Perhaps most importantly, water can improve muscle definition. When your muscles are overcome with drought, it is next-to-impossible to improve their appearance. Hydrated muscles are able to easily contract, boosting the power of your workouts and eliminating sagging skin.

Last, remember that your water consumption is most effective when spread throughout the course of the day. Also, it is not particularly healthy to "drown" your body's system by having too much water all at once. Instead, isolate three to four times daily where you know that you will have the time to enjoy a big glass of water and just sip water at other times throughout the day. And consider the fact that you should never let yourself become thirsty; when you are thirsty, you are already on your way to becoming dehydrated.

And what if you don't like water? That's okay; there are actually a lot of people who don't enjoy water. If you count yourself among those, try this: add a slice of lemon, lime, or other fruit in the glass you'll mimic the taste of your favorite soda without all the unhealthy effects. And if you really despise water, try drinking flavored water. However, be sure to read the label! Many so-called "healthy" sports drinks are filled with sugars, sodium, or chemicals.

So now you are ready to begin. Once you begin drinking your recommended daily water intake amount, you may be surprised to notice that your body almost immediately responds by decreasing your appetite—sometimes even on day number one. And if you are committed to becoming healthier, leaner, and happier (and of course you are, because you've read this far), water will become a vital, integral part of your day. It may just become one of the cornerstones of your weight-loss plan!

The Importance of Sleep

We all know that sleep is an absolutely critical part of our daily life. Unless we sleep enough every day, our bodies will collapse from exhaustion. Despite the essentiality of sleep, we vary widely in our sleep habits. In our 24/7 society, some of us can get away with four hours per night, although many of us are completely useless if we don't get nine hours every night. And besides our own personal preferences, our sleep requirements vary depending upon our familial, employment, and age-related requirements. However, what most of us don't know is that sleep is absolutely essential to not only to our level of alertness, but it also has a direct impact upon our health and weight-loss goals.

Some Facts to Consider

- Almost two-thirds of American adults (62 percent) experience some sort of problem sleeping *at least* several nights per week.
- Forty-three percent of American adults say they are so groggy during the day that it actually interferes with daily activities a few days per month or more.
- One out of five (20 percent) of American adults experience daytime sleepiness at least several days per week—or more.
- Almost one out of ten American adults (7 percent) admit to having changed jobs at some point in their lives in order to obtain more sleep.

How Much Sleep Is Enough for Me?

Ask average people if they're getting enough sleep and they'll tell you immediately, "Of course not." But if you ask those same people how much sleep they *actually require* to function optimally, their eyes will glaze over.

This is because each person's sleep requirement is different, and most of us simply haven't put the time in to find out how much we need. (In fact, some people may only need five or six hours of sleep to perform and work at their best; others may need nine, ten, or eleven hours to even feel decent). Studies have found that the average adult will function best with seven to eight hours of good nighttime sleep; yet, it is worthwhile to consider how much sleep you actually need.

Our sleep requirements are based directly upon "circadian rhythms," the inner biological clock that regulates our sleep and wake cycles. We have evolved to be "diurnal" animals (programmed to operate most effectively during daylight hours), as opposed to nocturnal (sleeping during the day and doing most of our activities at night). Please note that as infants, we are neither diurnal nor nocturnal and instead have sleep-wake cycles that are frequent and evenly spaced throughout every day.

For most adults, seven to eight hours a night appears to be the best amount of sleep. This is not just because a sound night's sleep puts us in a better mood or improves our concentration. Multiple studies have shown that adults who do not receive a minimal amount of sleep (less than six hours per night) actually have increased amounts of life-threatening diseases, such as diabetes. This is true for even the oldest of us who have long been considered to require less sleep. In fact, older adults are now known to actually get less sleep because of harmful sleep disruptions such as sleep apnea, pain, or arthritis, which can all shorten sleep periods (and which is exactly why many senior citizens need to nap during the day).

All sleep studies suggest that those adults who receive slightly over eight hours of undisturbed sleep once daily perform at optimum levels throughout the day. Of course, this will depend upon other factors, such as the quality of sleep obtained, stress levels, and overall health. It should be obvious, by now, that there are almost as many sleep patterns and sleep pattern preferences as there are people. It is critical that you take the time to find your own sleeping pattern that works for you not only for your peace of mind, but for your overall health and life expectancy! The following chapter will show you exactly why this is true.

Don't Let Your Weight-Loss Plans Be Sabotaged by Poor Sleeping Habits

Today, medical professionals and scientists agree: if you want to lose weight, proper sleep must be an essential part of your overall health plan.

Too Little Sleep = Too Much Overeating

Several studies have found a direct correlation between sleep and the hormones that influence our eating behaviors. There are two specific hormones involved: ghrelin, which is responsible for hunger pangs, and leptin, a hormone that tells the body when it is time to stop eating. When we are sleep-deprived, our bodies' ghrelin levels increase, while our leptin levels decrease, yielding the toxic mix of increased food cravings while simultaneously not feeling full. Further compounding this is the fact that when we are sleep-deprived, we tend to select different types of foods: most often high-calorie sweets, or salty, starchy carbs (which, as we know, are broken down into sugars). All of these bad habits, especially when applied together, will lead to long-term, substantial weight gain.

Find Your Optimal Sleep Pattern for Weight Loss

We stated earlier that it is advantageous for you to find how much sleep you need each night. "Fine," you say, "but how exactly should I do this?" To begin, try to sleep as long as you want for several days—which is probably best done during vacation (if you'd like to keep your job!). Within those few days, your sleep will stabilize: soon you will notice that you are waking up after the same number of hours of sleep each night (give or take twenty minutes.) When your sleep "stabilizes" like this, you have found your optimal sleep amount. Once you have determined how much sleep you actually need, make a plan. Get into a steady routine by setting a regular time to go to sleep each night and start getting ready ahead of time. (Sorry, but this means cutting out the TV or obsessing over work immediately before bed so that you'll be in the right frame of mind for sleeping.)

Sleep + Exercise + Healthy Eating = Weight Loss

While sleep is essential, don't overestimate the importance of sleep. Don't assume that taking a few extra hours of sleep each night will cause the pounds to just melt off! Exercising and eating healthfully are still the most important cornerstones of any healthy living plan, and getting enough sleep will just fortify these efforts.

However, lack of sleep is devastating, so much so that it is well on its way to being considered another obesity risk factor. If you have any doubts about this, consider the following: nearly two-thirds of all Americans are overweight, almost exactly the same number that researchers say are getting under eight hours of sleep each night. If you can practice just one item in this chapter, remember this: when our bodies are less hungry for sleep, they will be less hungry for food too.

The Rhythms of Eating and Sleeping Right

We mentioned circadian rhythms earlier, but equally important are our eating rhythms. This link between eating and sleeping is because of something known as our bodies' cortisol rhythm.

Maintaining A Normal Cortisol Rhythm: Critical for Sound Sleep

Produced by our bodies' adrenal glands (located directly above our kidneys), cortisol is a vital hormone in any effective weight-loss plan. Cortisol assists in regulating a host of bodily functions, such as: activating the thyroid hormone, bone resorption, muscle strength, energy production, resistance to infection, inflammation and autoimmune diseases, as well as regulation of allergic reactions. Additionally, cortisol is important in determining the potency of sleep's rejuvenating effects.

The hormone cortisol is produced cyclically, with the highest levels of release occurring in the morning. This twenty-four-hour cycle is part of the circadian rhythm. An abnormal circadian rhythm of adrenal hormones hurts many of the body's key functions, including immune surveillance and energy production. An upset of this rhythm results in the possibility of tiredness, easy bruising, infection, osteoporosis, low sex drive, infertility, migraine headaches, adult acne, bloating, and high blood pressure.

If your cortisol level is high overnight, you will have a negative impact on your rapid eye movement (REM) sleep. Hurting your REM sleep will result in waking up not refreshed, regardless of how many hours you may sleep. That is because REM sleep is the sleep stage where we have dreams, which is accompanied by a relaxation of the body and an increase in the rate of breathing. This intense dreaming is because of a heightened cerebral activity. The paralysis that occurs at the same time across all major muscle groups is considered by many to be a way to stop our bodies from physically acting out the powerful dreams that occur during this dynamic, intense sleep period.

For those of us who sleep over eight hours and still awake un-refreshed, REM-disrupted sleep is most likely the culprit. To have rejuvenating sleep, it is imperative that you have a normal cortisol level at night. The key to a normal nighttime cortisol level is a normal daytime cortisol rhythm.

The Link between the Glycemic Index and Cortisol

Our bodies' cortisol levels are highly (and rapidly) dependant on our food intake, so much so that a meal's glycemic index directly affects the cortisol level for up to five hours. As we discussed earlier, a food's glycemic index reflects how blood sugar level is affected by that food in question. Foods with high sugar and low fiber content have a high glycemic index. These foods yield wide variances in insulin levels, as compared to foods with low glycemic indexes. As we know through the study of diabetes, persistently high glucose levels exacerbate coronary artery disease. But of course, always consult your doctor before starting any weight loss program, and this is absolutely necessary if you are a diabetic.

Foods with a high glycemic index (or GI), including sugars, refined starches, and other highly processed foods, cause cortisol levels to rise. This is why those of us who start our day off with high-carb, starchy, or sugary breakfast (isn't this just about everyone?) automatically boost the blood's cortisol and force it to leave its normal level well behind. Unfortunately, this cortisol level often remains high all day and well into the night—which in turn makes the body "crash" and us begin looking for energy-boosters (often in the form of caffeine or more sugary foods) all over again. But even worse than having a high-GI meal is having no breakfast at all. Whenever we fast for more than five hours at a time, as we do overnight during sleep, our body's cortisol levels usually rise. And a rise above the normal range during daylight hours ensures that nighttime cortisol levels will also be high, thus disturbing REM sleep.

Always remember that just one late, skipped, or high-GI meal during the day will result in a high cortisol level at night. This high level of cortisol will carry over into night, ruin REM sleep, and replace it with furtive, restless sleep that does not properly refresh the body. However, low glycemic index foods—like meat, poultry, fish, vegetables, and other proteins—generally lower our cortisol levels. If you start the day with a normal cortisol level, then eating from a diet rich in the above-mentioned foods every three hours will keep our cortisol levels naturally trending downward.

The good news is that foods with high and low GI levels tend to balance each other out. Therefore, consuming high glycemic index foods like starch or grains requires an equal amount of low-GI foods, such as proteins. In general, on their own, vegetables are usually very well balanced regarding GI. To prevent rising levels of cortisol, we are best off balancing all sugars and grains (even whole grains) with animal protein. And if you do not consume animal protein for religious or socio-consciousness concerns, try to stick to more fruits and vegetables than a heavy carb diet, if possible. Too much of our food is overly-processed, overly-hydrogenated, and too high in GI.

The Effects of Non-Sprouted Grains on Cortisol

Today, because of hybridization due to processing, most of the grains we consume contain about half the protein they did nearly a century ago. Because most grains today are not given sufficient time to sprout when creating flour, most mass-produced breads and grains further disrupt our cortisol rhythm. That is because these non-sprouted grains create an inflammatory response in our stomach. This response forces the secretion of excess levels of cortisol into the intestinal tract. Because the gut is satiated with cortisol, other areas of the body are deprived of their normal allowance. As the rest of the body reacts to these depleted levels of cortisol with allergies and inflammation, the gut is besieged with abnormal amounts of bacteria, lowered immunity, and metabolic reactivity to foods. In fact, this reaction is so powerful that elevated nighttime cortisol suppresses the immune system—as well as our resistance to infection and cancer. Taking the time to sprout grains is so essential because sprouting removes many of the toxic peptides found on grains' hulls.

The Too-Many-Carbs Trap

If you have not been following the guidelines highlighted in this chapter, you may have already depleted the store of glycogen normally present in your liver. If so, you may often find yourself hypoglycemic in less than the (usual) five hours. If that is the case, it will normally take three months of regularly consuming glycemically balanced meals at regular intervals to replenish your liver's glycogen stores. This glycogen from the liver is essential to allowing our brains to function seamlessly during overnight (sleep time) fasting periods and any meals you may skip during daytime. Cortisol is so powerful, in fact, that our brains' cells are actually injured when glycogen is unavailable.

Be warned: one myth that has led to major health problems for many athletes is that foods high in sugar and starch help to promote glycogen storage. In fact, this "carb-loading" often leads many athletes to experience colossal fatigue and other conditions caused by depletion. Instead, balanced consumption of proteins, non-gluten grains, and non-fructose carbohydrates will counter this problem. As I detailed earlier, I have seen this problem with many Desi bodybuilders back home.

The Cortisol-Cancer Link

Besides disrupted REM sleep and throwing our bodies' processes out of whack, elevated nighttime cortisol levels actually suppress our immune systems. Unfortunately, this decreases our resistance to infection and even cancer. Multiple studies prove that elevated secretory midnight cortisol is directly correlated with an increased risk of breast cancer. Not surprisingly, people who correct their cortisol rhythm often report being better-protected against infections and disease.

Sex Hormone Balance and Cortisol

Just as our body can "steal" cortisol from the gut, it can also counteract abnormal cortisol levels by stealing from our sex hormones. Scientists named this "pregnenolone steal," because pregnenolone is a precursor of cortisol *and* our sex hormones. In short, abnormal cortisol yields derangements in our sex hormone balance. Imbalances of our sex hormones are extremely unhealthy. They can lead to a lowered sex drive, balding, prostate enlargement, urinary hesitancy, nighttime urination, PMS, uterine fibroids, heavy menstrual flow, and breast tenderness. Sex hormone imbalances are much easier to correct when our cortisol rhythm is normal. Likewise, with a chronic imbalance of the cortisol rhythm, long-lasting sex hormone balances are nearly impossible. Also note that hormone imbalances are not—contrary to public opinion—easily rectified just by taking more of whatever hormone is low. It is absolutely necessary that you determine *why* the particular hormone is low and directly address its root cause. The vast majority of times, it is necessary to fix any dietary shortfalls to safely replace and balance hormones.

A Note for Those with Naturally Occurring Abnormal Cortisol Rhythms

For the purpose of our discussion, we are assuming that you have a normal circadian rhythm of cortisol to begin with. If your rhythm naturally begins with disruption, you first need to correct the basic rhythm. Find a physician familiar with management of cortisol circadian rhythms. That being said, our circadian rhythm of cortisol can be disrupted from birth. Adding to this can be viral infections, trauma during birth (such as birth canal obstructions), an abnormal maternal rhythm, or irregular eating patterns. If the signals from the hypothalamus and pituitary glands to the adrenal glands are disrupted, an abnormal cortisol rhythm will result, regardless of sleep patterns.

Ouch! Pain Disrupts Cortisol, Too

Even basic pains, such as a headache or fever, can raise our cortisol level. In turn, this pain and its accompanying elevated cortisol add to the sleep disruption. In these cases, dietary adjustments alone are rarely enough; pain management and/or correction of the underlying causes are mandatory. And please note: even skipping or postponing a meal, or consuming a high-sugar/starch meal, can trip up your cortisol rhythm for the upcoming night—dramatically reducing the chance that the following day will start off on the right track, as far as a normal cortisol rhythm goes.

Yes, Emotions Affect Our Hormones, Too

Feeling threatened, or longing, will also release particular stress hormones, most notably cortisol. These emotions—including fear, frustration, anger, and sadness—simultaneously increase cortisol and reduce sex hormones. On top of these negative effects, digestive enzymes are not released during periods of extreme stress (also known as the "flight or fight" response.) During these times, food accumulates in the stomach and just decays instead of being digested, as is normal. That is because during these periods, the body concentrates all its actions on the "fight or flight" stimulus, producing adrenaline instead of digestive enzymes. In effect, our overall system asks our body, "Do I have enough of everything?" Today, in our modern society, the "fight or flight" reaction is common, but not for the basic primitive reasons we inherited from our forbearers.

Herbal Alternatives to Abnormal Cortisol

Whether you have abnormally high—or low—cortisol, you can adjust the levels naturally, via the use of herbs. If your level is too high, you may reduce it with herbs including de-glycerinized licorice (DGL), phosphorylated serine, or phosphatidyl serine. The latter of those three taken at 6:00 p.m. can assist in bringing a high cortisol level down to normal by bedtime. For some, this may take as little as an hour; in that case, you may need to take phosphorylated serine later in the evening.

If you have a cortisol level that is too low, you may want to try whole licorice root extract (*Glycyrrhiza glabra*): it does the opposite of DGL, raising the cortisol level. This herb is particularly beneficial for people with morning fatigue due to low cortisol. For these people, a cup of licorice tea in the morning can beat the lack of appetite often found by those with low cortisol levels.

The following tips will help.

How To Achieve a Normal, Balanced Cortisol Rhythm:

- Sleep at least eight hours.
- Eat breakfast within an hour of waking.
- Eat small, low glycemic index meals approximately every three hours while awake.
- Eat sprouted whole grains.
- As always, avoid sugars and starch as much as possible.
- Deal with pain. Don't allow it to fester; doing so will wreak havoc on your cortisol level.
- Combating emotional stress and following the first seven tips will ensure that you respond better to the day-to-day stresses of life.
- Speak with your physician regarding hormone function or therapies correcting cortisol rhythm (if needed).
- Meditate as much as possible. this will combat stress and allow your mind to turn off occasionally.

In conclusion, remember that reaching—and maintaining—a normal circadian rhythm of cortisol should be a priority. Normal cortisol rhythms are effective in fighting and warding off chronic infections, cancer, fatigue, and obesity; and can even dissipate a tendency to bruise easily, as well as stretch marks. In fact, if you deal with your cortisol rhythm and set it straight now, you may find yourself actually bounding out of bed in the morning (well, at least on the weekends). And as we all know, a positive attitude can never hurt your overall health.

The Importance of 5-HTP

The importance of sleep cannot be overstated: it is the time when our bodies repair, rebuild, and renew all the cells and compounds that have been damaged, drained, or otherwise depleted by the hazards of everyday life. 5-HTP is a compound that serves to promote healthier sleep cycles—and is now available in most health and fitness stores. 5-HTP, or L-5-Hydroxytryptophan is created when tryptophan in our body is converted into serotonin. 5-HTP is able to transverse the blood-brain barrier; it has been found to increase active serotonin levels and serotonin production. These increased serotonin levels are associated with healthier sleep, increased melatonin production for twenty-four-hour sleep cycle regulation, mood regulation, and better appetite control.

How 5-HTP Works

5-HTP is effective because it supports the balanced production of two essential sleep-regulating hormones: serotonin and melatonin. Serotonin, a neurotransmitter, assists in helping regulate moods, appetite, and sleep. However, we need sufficient levels serotonin in the first place to maintain these balances—which is where 5-HTP comes into place. 5-HTP is a precursor to serotonin, formed when tryptophan is converted into serotonin in our bodies. 5-HTP has been found to increase both the amount—and availability—of serotonin our bodies produce. 5-HTP crosses the blood-brain barrier, increasing serotonin blood levels and in our brain, helping the body to quickly, effectively regain a healthy balance during any time of the day, even during sleep.

This serotonin is eventually converted into melatonin. Melatonin is the hormone that regulates our circadian rhythms. Physical activity, emotional stress, and aging will decrease our melatonin levels, and upend our natural sleep cycle. But this balance can be regained with 5-HTP intake. When 5-HTP increases serotonin production, melatonin production is also increased, enabling even the most sleep-deprived of us to gain back healthier sleeping patterns as well as a well-balanced circadian rhythm. There are several brands of healthy, safe, and natural 5-HTP on the market today.

In Conclusion: Sleep Longer, Lower Your Stress, and Live Longer

When your alarm clock goes off each morning, do you find yourself wearing out the snooze button? Or do you actually jump out of bed looking forward to another new day? Although in our need-it-done-yesterday world many of us want to be in the second group, those who wake later have been found to have less stress. Truth is, there is actually a physiological difference between those of us who wake early and those who ride the snooze button. This is because cortisol, the body's principal stress hormone, varies depending upon the time we wake.

Remember that cortisol levels are controlled by the brain. During a stressful situation, this hormone will rise in production approximately fifteen to twenty minutes after the given incident. Also, our bodies produce varying levels of cortisol at different times throughout the day, regardless of stress and cortisol production is typically greater during the morning than at night. For the vast majority of us, this biological clock-based function contributes most to overall levels of cortisol and has a profound impact on our behavior and health. Scientists and doctors are only beginning to understand the vast array of ways stress impacts our well being. Recently, researchers have discovered that long exposure to high cortisol levels increases our risk for depression, degeneration of the brain, and decreased bone and muscle mass.

Additionally, cortisol levels are not affected just by how much sleep we get but at what time we arise. Although the early bird may enjoy a few advantages, including increased concentration or more energy early in the day, these same early risers were found to be more depressed, angrier, and more stressed toward nighttime. Those who take a little extra time to sleep in are continually found to be less stressed and possess sunnier dispositions. In closing, a multitude of factors determine our stress levels each day, and biological cortisol is just one of them. But if sleeping in an extra fifteen minutes or half-hour can make us more relaxed, this isn't exactly a difficult addition to our overall health plan, is it?

Vitamins and Minerals: What They Are and Their Importance to Your Diet

As Americans, we seem to be taking more vitamins and minerals than ever; as Desis, we may not be taking enough. Overall, as with many health matters, moderation is best. And with anything else, actually understanding what we are putting into our body is beneficial and critical to our good health. Before beginning, we will briefly discuss vitamins and minerals' place in our overall health.

Having the proper nutrition and diet sustains life, generates energy and promotes tissue growth and repair—and consists of these elements: 1) carbohydrates; 2) fat; 3) protein; 4) vitamins; 5) minerals; and 6) water. Carbs, fat, and proteins are called macronutrients. Our bodies need them in large amounts or energy-yielding nutrients. These macronutrients break down and provide your body with energy. Vitamins and minerals are micronutrients; your body requires them in small (but necessary) amounts. Micronutrients do not yield energy; they do assist your body in carrying out necessary physiological processes. And approximately forty of these nutrients are essential for life. Our bodies cannot manufacture our physiological needs. Therefore, our diet must offer the majority of these essential nutrients.

All vitamins fall into one of two categories: water—or fat-soluble. Water-soluble vitamins are excreted in urine; fat-soluble vitamins are stored in fat tissue. There are nine water-soluble vitamins: C and the eight B vitamins (thiamin, riboflavin, niacin, B6, B12, folate, biotin, and pantothenic acid); and four fat-soluble vitamins: A, D, E, and K. Each have unique roles and functions. For instance, Vitamin A improves eyesight; vitamin K helps blood clot.

Minerals fall into two categories: major or macronutrients and minor or trace nutrients. Macronutrients include calcium, phosphorus, potassium, sodium, chloride, magnesium, and sulfur. Micronutrients include iron, iodine, zinc, chromium, selenium, fluoride, molybdenum, copper, and manganese. Macronutrients require 100 mg per day; micronutrients are required in much smaller, trace amounts. Like their vitamin counterparts, these sixteen essential minerals play vital roles in your body.

Although each is critical, vitamins and minerals are different. Vitamins are organic; hence, they contain carbon, an element found in all life forms. However, minerals are purely inorganic elements. They are usually much simpler, chemically, than vitamins. Every vitamin is essential; your body only requires some minerals. Vitamins are affected by heat, light, and chemicals. Food preparation, processing, and storage must meet stringent guidelines to preserve your food's vitamins. However, minerals are less affected by food preparation. Yet mineral loss can occur when minerals are bound to other substances—oxalates found in spinach and tea or phytates in legumes and grains are examples—which makes them unavailable for your body's utilization.

As we mentioned, many Americans consume too much (or many) dietary supplements. Besides being costly, dietary supplements are often not enough to satisfy your body's nutritional requirements. Instead, garnering these nutrients from a wide-ranging diet complete with fresh fruits and vegetables is optimal.

Vitamins: Facts and Dosages

Vitamins are essential for our good health. They are found in many foods; the best way to meet these needs is by eating a well-balanced diet including many whole foods.

There are fifty-plus vitamins, minerals, and amino acids that help to keep you healthy. These many vitamins required by humans are similar because they are all made of the same few organic elements: carbon, hydrogen, oxygen, and occasionally nitrogen; B-12 also contains cobalt. Originally, these nutrients were classified as different because their elemental structures are each arranged differently. However, as scientific methods improved, one vitamin turned out to be in fact many vitamins. Vitamin B complex is the best example; it has many offshoots, like Vit B1,Vit B2,Vit B6,Vit B12, etc. However, some of these variations were found to be nonessential for humans; thus, we currently have gaps in the lists of subgroup letters and numbers. Today to ease confusion there are only thirteen true, essential vitamins. To stress their importance, the US government has instituted the Recommended Daily Allowance, or RDA, for each of the eighteen total essential vitamins and minerals. Established to serve as a goal for good nutrition, this information may be found on all American foods and beverages.

Each one of the thirteen essential vitamins performs at least one specific beneficial function for our body. When any one is missing, a deficiency disease may manifest. Vitamins do not provide energy, and they do not construct or build any part of the body, yet they are required for transforming foods into energy and body maintenance. Many studies have determined that consuming the proper levels of essential vitamins is necessary for life. Conversely, your body has no need for any excess vitamins ingested. In fact, overdoses of some vitamins can even be fatal (or at the least, dangerous). Additionally, your body can only store some vitamins for relatively short periods of time. For example: A, D, E, and K are absorbed with fat from foods and are stored in the body; water-soluble vitamins (the B's and C's) are typically not stored and are excreted in urine.

Vitamin Daily Allowance	General Information	*Deficiency Diseases*	Food Source
Vitamin A (Retinol) Men 600 mcg Women 600 mcg Children 600 mcg Infants 350 mcg Lactating Women 950 mcg	Vitamin A (Retinol) stimulates vision in the retina, prevents eye diseases, helps digestion of protein and secretion of gastric fluids. It is required for reproduction and growth.	Night-blindness and Keratomalacia, acne, boils, premature wrinkles, poor vision, night-blindness	Liver (beef, chicken, turkey, fish), carrots, broccoli leaves, sweet potatoes, kale, butter, spinach, leafy vegetables, pumpkin, collard greens, cantaloupe melon, eggs, apricots, papaya, mango, peas, broccoli, winter squash

Vitamin B1 (Thiamine) Men 1.3 mg Women 1.0 mg Children 1.1 mg Infants 50 mcg	Vitamin B1 (Thiamine) aids digestion of carbohydrates, promotes growth, stimulates brain function, protects the heart muscle, and regulates normal functioning of the nervous system.	Beriberi, Wernicke-Korsakoff syndrome, poor digestion, loss of weight, mental depression, and insomnia.	Wholegrain cereals, especially wheat, rice, and oats. Capsicum, turnip greens, apricots, pineapples, pistachio nuts, sheep liver, and mutton.
Vitamin B2 (Riboflavin) Men 1.5 mg Women 1.2 mg Children 1.3 mg Infants 60 mcg	Vitamin B2 (Riboflavin) metabolizes carbohydrates, fats, and proteins, prevents constipation, and promotes a healthy skin, nails, and hair.	Ariboflavinosis, oily hair, oily skin, premature wrinkles, split nails, anemia, vaginal itching, and cataracts.	Turnip greens, beets, radish leaves, colocasia and carrot leaves, papaya, raisins, custard, apples, and apricots; sheep liver and eggs, cow's milk, almonds, walnuts, pistachio nuts, and mustard seeds.

Vitamin B3 (Niacin) Men 17 mg Women 13 mg Children 15 mg Infants 650 mcg	Vitamin B3 (Niacin) helps metabolize proteins and carbo-hydrates and regula-tion the function of the gastro-intestinal tract. Dilates the blood capillary system, helps regu-lates proper blood circulation and the functioning of the nervous system. It is also essential for synthesis of estrogen, progesterone, and testosterone, as well as cortisone, thyrox-in, and insulin.	Pellagra, sores in the mouth, irri-tability, ner-vousness, skin lesions, diarrhea, forgetful-ness, insom-nia, chronic headaches, digestive disorders, and anemia.	Sheep liver, lean meats, prawns, cow's milk, rice, wheat, groundnuts, sunflower seeds, al-monds, turnip, beet greens, and the leaves of carrots and celery.

Vitamin B1 (Thiamine) Men 1.3 mg Women 1.0 mg Children 1.1 mg Infants 50 mcg	Vitamin B1 (Thiamine) aids digestion of carbohydrates, promotes growth, stimulates brain function, protects the heart muscle, and regulates normal functioning of the nervous system.	Beriberi, Wernicke-Korsakoff syndrome, poor digestion, loss of weight, mental depression, and insomnia.	Wholegrain cereals, especially wheat, rice, and oats. Capsicum, turnip greens, apricots, pineapples, pistachio nuts, sheep liver, and mutton.
Vitamin B2 (Riboflavin) Men 1.5 mg Women 1.2 mg Children 1.3 mg Infants 60 mcg	Vitamin B2 (Riboflavin) metabolizes carbohydrates, fats, and proteins, prevents constipation, and promotes a healthy skin, nails, and hair.	Ariboflavinosis, oily hair, oily skin, premature wrinkles, split nails, anemia, vaginal itching, and cataracts.	Turnip greens, beets, radish leaves, colocasia and carrot leaves, papaya, raisins, custard, apples, and apricots; sheep liver and eggs, cow's milk, almonds, walnuts, pistachio nuts, and mustard seeds.

| Vitamin B3 (Niacin) Men 17 mg Women 13 mg Children 15 mg Infants 650 mcg | Vitamin B3 (Niacin) helps metabolize proteins and carbo-hydrates and regula-tion the function of the gastro-intestinal tract. Dilates the blood capillary system, helps regu-lates proper blood circulation and the functioning of the nervous system. It is also essential for synthesis of estrogen, progesterone, and testosterone, as well as cortisone, thyrox-in, and insulin. | Pellagra, sores in the mouth, irri-tability, ner-vousness, skin lesions, diarrhea, forgetful-ness, insom-nia, chronic headaches, digestive disorders, and anemia. | Sheep liver, lean meats, prawns, cow's milk, rice, wheat, groundnuts, sunflower seeds, al-monds, turnip, beet greens, and the leaves of carrots and celery. |

Vitamin Daily Allowance	General Information	Deficiency Diseases	Food Source
Vitamin B5 (Pantothenic acid) Men 10 mg Women 10 mg Children 5.5 mg	Vitamin B5 (Pantothenic acid) metabolizes carbohydrates, fats, and proteins, synthesis of amino acids and fatty acids. Helps with formation of porphyrin, which is found in the hemoglobin of the red blood cells. It stimulates the adrenal glands and increases production of cortisone and other adrenal hormones.	Paresthesia, chronic fatigue, mental depression, dizziness, and muscular weakness.	Yeast, liver, eggs, peanuts, mushrooms, split peas, soya beans, and soya bean flour.
Vitamin B6 (Pyridoxine) Men 2.0 mg Women 2.0 mg Children 1.7 mg Infants 0.1-0.4 mg	Vitamin B6 (Pyridoxine) metabolizes fats, and proteins, prevents nervous and skin disorders, provides protection against a high cholesterol level, certain types of heart disease, and diabetes.	Anemia, edema, mental depression, skin disorders, nervousness, eczema, and kidney stones.	Yeast, sunflower seeds, wheat germ, soya beans, walnuts, lentils, and lima beans

Vitamin B8 (Biotin) Men 100-200 mcg Women 100-200 mcg Children 50-200 mcg Infants 35 mcg	Vitamin B8 (Biotin) metabolizes carbo-hydrates, fats, and proteins. It is involved with health of hair, skin, and nails.	Dermatitis, enteritis, muscular weakness, pains, las-situde, lack of appetite, eczema, dandruff, hair loss and sebor-rhea.	Brewer's yeast, beef liver, rice bran, rice germ, rice polishings, and peanut butter.

Vitamin B9 (Folic acid) Men 100 mcg Women 100 mcg Children 80 mcg Infants 25 mcg Pregnant Women 400 mcg Lactating Women 150 mcg	Vitamin B9 (Folic acid) is important for growth and division of all body cells, produces nucleic acids, RNA (ribonucleic acid) and DNA (deoxyribonucleic acid), aids in protein metabolism, and contributes to normal growth. Helps in the building of antibodies that prevent and heal infections.	Anemia, skin disorders, loss of hair, impaired circulation, a grayish-brown skin pigmentation, fatigue, and mental depression.	Bulses, legumes, cluster beans, spinach, mint, gingelly seeds, and meat.

| Vitamin B12 (Cyanocobalamin) Men 2 mcg Women 2 mcg Children 1 mcg Infants 0.5 mcg Lactating Women 2.6 mcg | Vitamin B12 (Cyanocobalamin) is necessary for proper utilization of fats, carbohydrates, and proteins for body building, helps produce and regenerate red blood cells, improves concentration, memory, and balance, and relieves irritability. | Megaloblastic anemia, chronic fatigue, a sore mouth, a feeling of numbness or stiffness, loss of mental energy, and difficulty in concentration. | Meat, liver, eggs, shrimp, and dairy. |

Vitamin Daily Allowance	General Information	Deficiency Diseases	Food Source
Vitamin C (Ascorbic acid) Men 40 mg Women 40 mg Children 40 mg Infants 25 mg Lactating Women 80 mg	Vitamin C (Ascorbic acid) helps formation of collagen, enhances the absorption of iron, vitality, endurance, clear skin, healthy gums, and teeth. It is involved in the vital functions of all glands and organs, maintenance of bones and proper functioning of the adrenal and thyroid glands.	Scurvy, soft gums, skin hemorrhages, capillary weakness, deterioration in collagen, anemia, and slow heating of sores and wounds.	Gooseberries, guavas, limes, lemons, oranges, papayas, citrus fruits, and vegetables
Vitamin D (Calciferol) Men 0.01 mg Women 0.01 mg Children 0.01 mg	Vitamin D (Calciferol) helps assimilation of calcium, phosphorus, and other minerals in the digestive tract. Is important for healthy functioning of the parathyroid glands, which regulate the calcium level in the blood and proper formation of teeth and bones.	Rickets, Osteomalacia. Can cause muscular weakness, lack of vigor, deficient assimilation of minerals, pyorrhea, brittle or soft bones, and retarded growth.	Sunlight— ten to fifteen minutes of sunlight a day.

Vitamin E (Tocopherol) Men 15 mg Women 12 mg Children 8.3 mg Infants 4-5 mg	Vitamin E (Tocopherol) oxygenates the tissues, is essential for fertility, prevents unsaturated fatty acids, sex hormones, and fat-soluble vitamins from being destroyed in the body by oxygen. Helps prevention of heart disease, asthma, arthritis, and many other conditions.	Spinocerebellar ataxia and myopathies.	Wheat germ oil, sunflower oil, almond oil, hazelnuts, walnut oil, peanut oil, olive oil, peanuts, pollard, corn, asparagus, oats, chestnuts coconut, tomatoes, carrots, goat's milk
Vitamin K (Phylloquinone) Men 70-140 mcg Women 70-140 mcg Children 35-75 mcg	Vitamin K (Phylloquinone) prevention of internal bleeding and hemorrhages, important for the normal functioning of the liver, and helps with energy-producing activities of the tissues, particularly those of the nervous system.	Bleeding diathesis.	Cauliflower, cabbage, spinach, alfalfa, yogurt, soy beans.

How Vitamins Work

The idea that vitamins can replace food is a common misconception. Actually, vitamins cannot be assimilated without the ingestion of food. For this reason, we suggest that you always take your vitamins at mealtime.

Vitamins are known to assist in regulating metabolism, converting fat and carbs into energy, and helping to form **Error! Hyperlink reference not valid.** and tissue. Vitamins are now recognized as having a critical role to play in your most basic nutritional needs. In fact, in 1996, the Food and Drug Administration (FDA) created regulations requiring the addition of folic acid to corn meals, cereals, enriched breads, flours, pastas, rice, and other grains. This regulation was an answer to the discovery that thousands of American babies were born each year with spina bifida because their moms were not receiving enough folate in their diets. (Spina bifida is an often-fatal neural tube defect occurring in pregnancy's first month when the spinal column does not entirely close.) The government initiated the introduction of folate into these goods since many Americans eat flour products and likewise do not get enough leafy green vegetables (which contain folate) and has since saved thousands of lives.

However, today many healthcare professionals advocate a more far-ranging course of supplement requirements and recognize that vitamin supplements play an important role in our nutrition. To achieve and maintain proper health, many believe that there are in fact over forty essential micronutrients (vitamins, minerals, and other bio-nutrients)—and often, diet alone is not enough to provide these.

Vitamins and Minerals: Their Roles

Vitamins are essential to good health, and many have critical roles to play. Vitamin A, for example, aids in developing and maintaining body tissues like bone and skin. And it also improves vision, nervous system functioning, reproduction, and growth. The range of B vitamins increase production of fats, proteins, and carbs and helps with metabolism, building red blood cells, and maintaining the nervous system's protective covering. Vitamin C helps to form tissues, cells, bones, and teeth; heals wounds; and boosts immune system performance. Vitamin E protects the outer cell membranes—which then helps your immune system stave off diseases. Meanwhile, Vitamin K helps blood clot in wounds.

Minerals, too, have wide-ranging functions; up to twenty play significant roles in your body. Micro-minerals, those that your body only requires traces of, are powerful enough to fight serious illness; included here are copper, iodine, chromium, iron, fluorine, tin, zinc, nickel, vanadium, manganese, silicon, molybdenum, and selenium. Macro-minerals—those which the body needs large amounts of—include magnesium, sodium, potassium, chlorine, phosphorus, calcium, and sulfur. Zinc helps metabolize proteins and keeps enzymes functioning properly. Enzymes require copper to thoroughly metabolize. Iodine is required to keep the thyroid working properly. Calcium (and phosphorus) builds strong bones and teeth. Iron delivers needed oxygen to cells. Potassium aids muscle contraction, cells' fluid balance, and transmittal of messages through the body's nerves and keeps the kidneys and heart working correctly.

Not only do vitamins and minerals help the body function, but they also strengthen each other. For example, the body absorbs iron with vitamin C's help. Vitamin D helps the absorption of phosphorus and calcium. Likewise, vitamins D and K are the only vitamins the body can supply itself. Your skin creates vitamin D when exposed to sunlight; K is produced by intestinal bacteria. Yet, outside sources must supply our bodies with all other vitamins.

The Two Categories of Vitamins

Vitamins are divided into two categories and are classified according to the substance that carries them throughout the body.

Water-soluble vitamins are carried throughout the body in water; they need daily replacement because they are lost in body fluids, such as sweat and urine. These include folacin (folic acid), biotin, pantothenic acid, thiamin (B1), riboflavin (B2), niacin (B3), pyridoxine (B6), and cyanocobalamin (B12). Fat-soluble vitamins are carried by fats located in the bloodstream, and include A (retinol), D (calciferol), E (d-alpha-tocopherol), and K (menaquinone). Fats are stored better than water; thus when intake of fat-soluble vitamins is disrupted, it is less critical than when water-soluble vitamins are interrupted. Regardless, when extremes of either vitamin-type are taken, they can quickly reach toxic levels.

Vitamin and Minerals as Supplements

Vitamins and minerals are a six-billion-dollar-a-year industry in America; studies have shown that nearly three-quarters of all Americans take at least one. However, vitamins should not be used as substitutions for a healthy diet—but instead as a supplement. In general, whenever possible, it is advisable to eat vitamins in their food variety and in pill form, despite their beneficial effects, because dietitians worry that people will begin to use them instead of healthy eating habits.

However, this fact does not address the pure severity of the health crisis in America, let alone Desi lands. The vast majority of Americans do not eat ideal diets. In fact, over half of all Americans do not drink a glass of juice, consume one serving of vegetables, or eat one piece of fruit daily. In fact, only 40 percent eat three to five servings of vegetables daily, the recommended amount—and only 20 percent eat the recommend two to four servings of fruit each day. Regardless of what the healthcare professionals wish, for the many people who are not eating properly, supplementation is better than nothing, at least.

Vitamins and Nutritional Supplements

People who get enough vitamins by eating a varied diet do not need to take a vitamin. However, as we stated, this does not include the vast majority of Americans, let alone in the Desi culture. For those who do not eat a varied diet, may become deficient in some vitamins. This is particularly so for the elderly, who often do not eat enough different kinds of food and may benefit from a vitamin supplement.

Multiple studies suggest that the body uses up more vitamins when it is under stress, including stress caused by illness and daily routines. Thus, many people therefore take vitamins when they are busy, feeling run down, or at the first signs of a cold coming on. Smoking will make it harder for the body to absorb vitamins, so if you do happen to smoke, you should either pay special attention to your diet or take a vitamin supplement or both. Of course, it goes without saying that quitting smoking altogether is always the best option.

The Desi Diet Recipes

The problem with Desi food, as we discussed in our introduction, is not the food itself but rather the way in which it is (most often) cooked. Desi food does include plenty of vegetables and whole grains, such as lentils and legumes. However, the fact that Desi foods, even healthy ones, are often deep-fried removes all their inherent nutritional value.

The majority of calories and nutritional value in Desi foods depend on the way in which they are cooked. As a rule, a dish will be very high in calories, mostly from fat, if it has been deep-fried. Conversely, the very same dish can be low in calories and fat and be perfectly healthy if it is steamed, stir-fried, or baked. In general, rich, creamy foods slathered in spice-colored liquids are high in fat and mostly saturated fat, the worst kind. On the other hand, tandoori dishes (cooked in a cyndrical clay oven, over coal or wood) are much more healthy and low in fat. Desis also have some peculiar eating habits that contribute to the unhealthiness of our foods. Desis tend to often reheat and overheat a lot of our food, which can destroy the food's nutrients.

In regard to India, northern dishes are usually rich in taste and presentation as compared to their southern neighbors. North Indian foods, particularly Punjabi, are often higher in calories and fat and lower in nutritional value, than south Indian foods. Northern meals and especially Punjabi cooking uses *tarka or vaghar* (frying of spices, onions, etc.) in straight ghee (which is high in saturated fats), butter, oil, trans fats, or trans-fatty acids (including hydrogenated oils and fats), which accounts for that unique Indian taste and texture.

North India's tandoori foods are rich in nutrition and natural flavors but are often filled with fats. As compared to American health foods, which are notoriously fat-laden, certain tandoori favorites are even worse.

Trans-fatty acids in:

- French fries: 4.2 percent–6.1 percent
- *Bhatura*: 9.5 percent
- *Paratha*: 7.8 percent
- *Puri* and *Aloo tikki*: 7.6 percent

Keeping the Good in Desi food

As we mentioned, the health benefits of Desi food are directly interrelated with its method of cooking. When a recipe calls for excessive cream, yogurt, ghee, or oil, usually with crushed cashews, the dish will be rich-tasting but low in nutritional value. North Indian foods, Punjabi foods, and those available in most Desi restaurants are typically overcooked like this and thus are higher in fat and lacking nutritionally. Additionally, these foods are often prepared with deep fried onions, ginger, and spices in oil or ghee. To counter our Desi cooking tendencies, we offer the following tips:

1. **Never deep-fry:** Instead, stir fry or sauté your meal in a bit of vegetable oil. Overcooked foods lose their nutritional value because vitamins, minerals, and other nutrients are leached out by the frying. And for vegetables, you should always stop cooking while the vegetable is still crisp to the touch.

2. **Avoid trans-fat altogether:** In Desi culture that means *no dalda vanaspati ghee, rath ghee, etc.,* for cooking. Also, watch out, because many restaurants and shops use trans-fats for cooking *aloo tikki, bhaturas, parathas, puri (poori)* and even sweets and vegetable curries. When in doubt, ask.

3. **Don't chop vegetables into very small pieces:** The more exposed surfaces a vegetable has, the more it will lose its nutrients because of exposure to the atmosphere.

4. **Chop vegetables *as* you cook them:** Don't chop vegetables and then allow them to sit (for the same reasons as number three, above).

5. **Do not wash vegetables after chopping:** Spinach, zucchini, lauki, etc. Chopping and washing further strips nutrients. Wash these vegetables before chopping them.

6. **Never overheat oil when you stir-fry:** It further breaks down nutritional values.

7. **When making pakoras, keep your besan batter thick:** Remember, when you deep-fry thin batter like besan, the pakoras absorb too much oil.

8. **Never add ghee or oil when making dough for poori:** If you do, the pooris will absorb too much oil while they are frying.

If you follow the guidelines above, you will be able to recreate a modern, healthier version of all the Desi dishes and entrees you love from your childhood. By being careful of your cooking methods and fat use, you will create tasty dishes with less fat—while keeping our culture's natural nutrition values and low calories.

A Few Words Regarding Curry

Curry comes from the Tamil word *kari* and means sauce. Curry has also come to refer to vegetables or meat eaten with *roti, chapati, naan, papadum,* and rice. India and many South Asian countries are known for their first-rate curries. Common varieties include vegetable, *mattar-paneer,* potato, beans, *kofta, korma, vindaloo,* chicken, *mutton,* and Rogan Josh curries. Typical curries include ghee, yogurt, and multiple spices: turmeric, red chili and/or coriander powder, cumin seed, mustard seed, and ginger. The subtle blending of these spices gives each dish its particular flavor, texture, and taste. A curry may be mild or hot, depending on the amount of spices used to prepare a given dish. However, when too much oil is used—particularly those like ghee—the curry will be too high in fat and calories.

While the wrong oils and poor cooking methods can have negative effects on the nutritional value of our meals, conversely, vegetables have a myriad of positive effects. Vegetables in our Desi culture help regulate high blood pressure and can lower cholesterol. Following our guidelines above, each vegetable recipe in this chapter preserves the valuable nutritional effects of the vegetable while remaining low-fat or fat-free. Our recipes shun ghee, instead opting for oils (vegetable oils, mainly) that are low in unhealthy saturated fats.

This section contains some wonderful vegetable curry recipes. Each dish is tasty, tempting, and nutritious; you'll think you're back in your homeland. Unlike typical Indian, Pakistani, or other South Asian restaurants, the curry dishes in the *Desi Diet* are low in fat and moderate in calories.

Menu Overviews and Recipes

Vegetarian Food

Desi vegetarian recipes are, simply put, life-prolonging sustenance. Regularly eating the foods in this section and shunning those high in fats, sodium, cholesterol, and sugars will check your cholesterol and high blood pressure and reduce risk for heart disease, diabetes, and obesity.

Desi Whole Grains

Whole grains, legumes, and lentils are rich in complex carbohydrates, protein, and dietary fiber. Additionally, whole pulses contain soluble and insoluble fibers. Because of the presence of complex carbs, these foods are digested and absorbed slowly and burned off by the body over time, *not* deposited as fat, like simple carbs tend to be.

"Whole grains" refer to grains' edible parts and include all three layers intact: the inner (germ), middle (endosperm), and outer (bran). The germ and bran provide vitamins E and B and minerals including zinc, selenium, copper, iron, manganese, and magnesium. These whole grains also contain phytochemicals, lignans, and antioxidants—potent weapons in warding off disease and illness. Milling whole grains removes their bran and germ, leaving only endosperm, a starch. Whole grains include wheat, rice, corn, grams, and oats. Whole-meal bread, pasta, and cereals contain whole grains, with oats, barley, and rye being particularly rich in soluble fiber.

Whole cereals are a particularly good source of dietary fiber, vitamins, proteins, and minerals. Also, they are low in fat. True whole grain cereals, in fact, can provide most of our body's energy demands. Yet, sadly, a significant portion of protein and other healthy elements are lost during refining. For example, white flour has little to no nutritional value; it is simply refined cereal produced from whole wheat that has had the majority of its germ and bran stripped.

Since whole grains are rich in dietary fiber, vitamins, and minerals, with little fat or cholesterol, they have been deemed "heart-friendly." Additional minerals, including magnesium, further prevent heart disease; too little magnesium in our diet has been known to foster high blood pressure and heart attacks.

Americans and Desis rarely eat whole grains. Traditionally, in the United States, anyway, we have tended to buy white bread. Nowadays, we have been conned into purchasing breads marked "rye," "pumpernickel," "multi-grain," "stone-ground," and "oatmeal" breads. In fact, these breads are all highly-processed, sugar-laden white bread variations (dishonestly) passed off as whole grains. This is a shame, because *whole grains can actually protect your heart and may reduce the risk of colon, mouth and stomach cancers.*

As always, be a label-reader. Always try to buy bread with the "whole grain" label, preferably with whole grain as its first ingredient. *But* be wary of any bread label that includes the words "high fructose corn syrup," "bleached," "enriched," or "refined." These words mean that the bread has in fact been processed and is not a true whole grain. According to the website of the Whole Grains Council, the symbol on the product's label indicates whole grain content-level:

- **100 percent/Excellent Source:** the product contains at least sixteen grams of whole grain per labeled serving and no refined grains
- **Excellent Source:** contains at least sixteen grams of whole grain per labeled serving
- **Good Source:** contains at least eight grams of whole grain per labeled serving
- **Wheat flour:** contains only 25 percent whole wheat flour

How Much Whole Grain Is Enough?

Ideally, you should consume three or more servings of whole grains per day. (One serving is one slice of whole wheat bread, half a whole wheat muffin, or half a cup of any of cooked oatmeal, whole wheat pasta, polenta, or brown rice).

Many of the whole grain recipes in this chapter are vegetarian; all are healthy. And all preserve the ingredients' nutritional value and are low-fat. The recipes are all ghee-free and use oils that are low in saturated fat and high in monounsaturated and polyunsaturated fats, including oils like olive, canola, or vegetable.

Desi Breads

There are various Desi breads, including *roti, chapatti, phulka,* or *naan.* Desi breads are made of whole wheat flour and typically cooked on a flat pan or *tave.* However, *naan* is made of plain flour *(maida)* and is cooked in a *tandoor* oven. *Chapati* or *roti* are eaten daily in North India; *naan* is typical of Punjab. South Indians eat *roti* only on occasion; restaurants serve *roti* and *naan,* but *naan* is the more popular choice.

Baking Roti and Chapati

Rolling *roti* and their cooking is something of an art form. This begins with rolling with a rolling pin; the *roti* rotates over and over on the rolling plate, continually growing in size. To make an excellent *roti,* the wheat dough should be prepared in advance, by at least thirty minutes.

- To begin, heat a *tava* (frying pan) on your stovetop, on medium heat.
- Once the *tava* is hot, put the roti on it; after three to four minutes (depending on your stove), the *roti* will be half-cooked.
- Flip the *roti* over and cook for an additional five to seven minutes.
- Flip it again, and press the *roti* gently with a cloth, allowing it to pop up. (You may also remove the *tava* and put the *roti* directly on the flame.)
- This process will transform the *roti* into a small popped-up, flying saucer shape.

Just one reminder: Avoid very fine flour. Fine flour lacks fiber. Also, do not sieve the flour; this process removes all the flour's remaining fiber.

Other types of Desi bread are listed and described below:

Desi Breads	
Name of Bread	**Description**
Roti, Chappati	Cooked on *tava,* a thin, round shape bread of wheat flour
Tandoori Roti	Baked in a *Tandoor,* a thick, round bread of wheat flour
Naan	Baked, thick oval bread of plain flour (*maida*)
Puri, Kachori	Deep-fried small puffed bread of wheat flour
Paratha	Shallow-fried thick round, square, or triangular bread
Tandoori Paratha	Baked in *Tandoor;* thick, oval-shaped bread stuffed with lentils, potato, or other filling
Stuffed *Paratha*	Shallow-fried, thick, round, square, or triangular bread stuffed with lentils, potato, or other filling
Bhatura	Deep-fried, thick, round bread made of plain flour (*maida*)

Desi Desserts

Desi sweets are generally based upon *khoya, mawa* (highly-thickened milk), *paneer* (cottage cheese), and *besan (*chickpea flour.) Additionally, sugar and *gur jaggery* are used to sweeten almost all Desi desserts. Garnishing is common, with almond, cardamom, pistachios, watermelon seeds, raisin, saffron, and rosewater being favorites. Popular delicacies include rasgulla, jalebi, laddu, and halwa.

Weights and Measures
1 Ounce = 30 ML = ⅛ Cup
2 Ounces = 60 ML = ¼ Cup
4 Ounces = 120 ML - ½ Cup
8 Ounces = 240 ML = 1 Cup 16 Ounces = 1 Pint = 2 Cups
32 Ounces = 1 Quart = 4 Cups
1 Liter = 1000 ML = 4 Cups (Approx)
1 Gallon = 128 Ounces = 16 Cups
1 Teaspoon = 5 ML
1 Tablespoon = 15 ML
2 Tablespoon = 1 Ounce
8 Tablespoons = 4 Ounces = ½ Cup
16 Tablespoons = 8 Ounces = 1 Cup
1 Pound = 455 Grams
1 Pound = 16 Ounces
2.2 Pounds = 1 Kg
1 Cup Sugar = 6 Ounces
1 Cup Water = 8 Ounces
1 Cup Plain Flour = 4 Ounces
1 Cup Rice = 7.5 Ounces
1 Cup Almonds = 5 Ounces
1 Cup Barley = 7 Ounces
1 Cup Beans = 7 Ounces
1 Cup Breadcrumbs = 2 Ounces
1 Cup Figs = 6 Ounces
1 Cup Milk = 8.25 Ounces
1 Cup Oats (Rolled) = 2.75 Ounces
1 Cup Peanuts = 6.25 Ounces
1 Cup Prunes = 5 Ounces

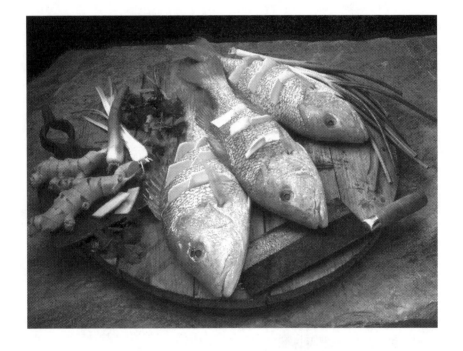

Achari Machli Steak

Serves 4–6

Ingredients:

4 thick fish steaks (swordfish, salmon, tuna, etc.)
2 red chilies, chopped
2 green chilies, chopped
1-inch piece ginger root, sliced
5 curry leaves
Juice of 4 lemons
2 garlic cloves, crushed
1 onion, chopped
4 tbsp. vegetable oil
½ tsp. ground turmeric
1 tbsp. ground coriander
2/3 cup pickling vinegar
1 tbsp. granulated sugar
Salt, to taste
½ tomato and salad leaves to garnish

Mix lemon juice, ginger, garlic, and chilies in a large bowl. Pat steaks dry and rub mixture on all sides of fish. Cover and marinate three hours in refrigerator.

Next, heat oil in large frying pan and sauté onion, turmeric, curry leaves, and coriander until the onion softens. Add the fish steaks to the onion mixture and fry for five minutes and then turn them over. Add the vinegar, sugar, and salt and bring to a boil. Lower the heat and simmer until fish is fully cooked. Transfer fish to serving platter, spooning onion mixture over them. Chill for twenty-four hours before serving, garnishing with salad leaves and tomato.

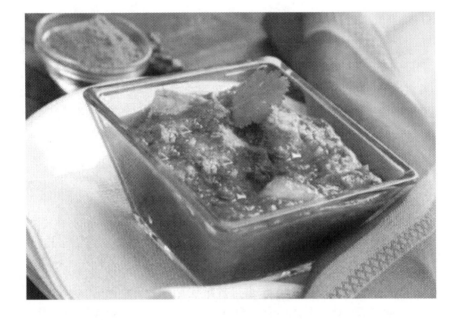

Tuna Fish Curry
Serves 4

Ingredients:

14-ounce can tuna in brine, drained
1 onion, sliced
1 green bell pepper, sliced
1 red bell pepper, sliced
2 garlic cloves, crushed
1 green chili, chopped
1-inch piece grated root ginger
2 tbsp. coriander, chopped
2 tbsp. vegetable oil
1 tsp. lemon juice
¼ tsp. garam masala
¼ tsp. cumin seeds
½ tsp. ground cumin
½ tsp. ground coriander
½ tsp. chili powder
¼ tsp. salt
Coriander springs, as garnish
Pita bread (warmed) and cucumber raita, to serve

Heat oil in large pan or wok and stir-fry cumin seeds until they start to sputter. Add ground cumin, coriander, chili powder, and salt. Cook for two to three minutes and then add garlic, onion, and peppers. Fry for five to seven minutes or until the onion browns.

Next, stir in tuna, green chili, and ginger and cook for five minutes. Add masala, lemon juice, and chopped coriander. Continue cooking for three to four minutes and serve in warm pita bread pockets with the cucumber raita. Garnish with coriander sprigs.

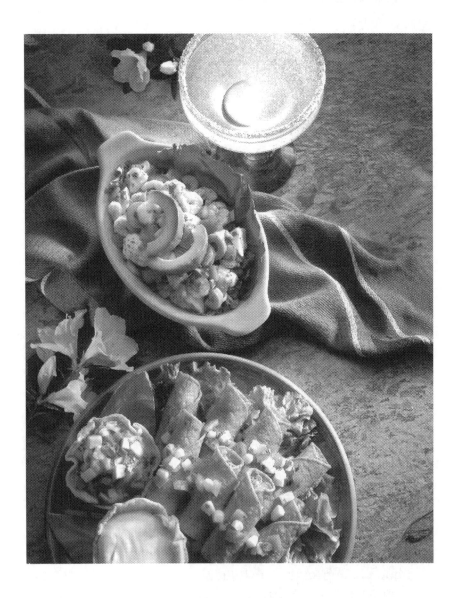

Fish Singapuri
Serves 4

Ingredients:

4 redfish, black bream or porgy, about 10 ounces each.
1 French loaf
1 mango
1 tbsp. vegetable oil
6 ounces baby spinach
½-inch ginger root, grated finely.
1 red chili, chopped
2 tbsp. lime juice
2 tbsp. chopped coriander
5 ounces bok choy
6 ounces cherry tomatoes, halved

Preheat oven to 350 degrees Fahrenheit. Cut the French loaf lengthwise and then slice into thick pieces. Bake for fifteen minutes. Meanwhile, prepare grill or preheat broiler. Deeply score both sides of fish and lightly moisten with oil. Grill or broil for six minutes, turning once.

Peel mango and slice one half, setting aside. Place other half in food processor, with ginger, mango, chili, lime juice, and coriander. Process on a low setting until smooth. Add water until mixture can be poured, about two to three tbsp.

Wash spinach and bok choy, patting dry with paper towel. Place fish on layer of leaves, spooning mango dressing on top. Garnish with reserved mango slices and tomato halves. Serve with French bread.

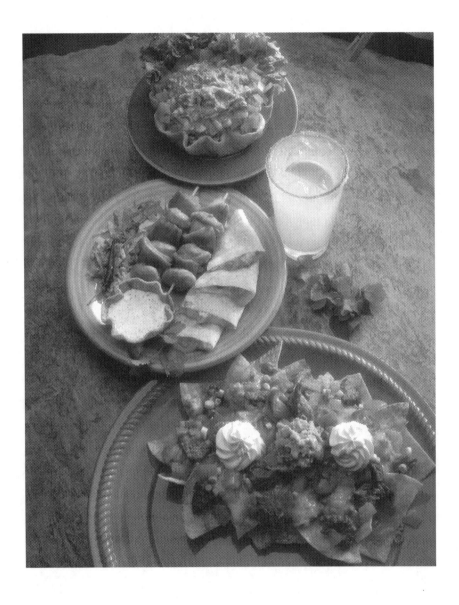

Venison Masala
Serves 4

Ingredients:

1 pound diced venison
1/3 cup split red lentils
4 tbsp. corn oil
2 green chilies, chopped
2 medium tomatoes, quartered
2 cloves
4 whole black peppercorns
1 tbsp. coriander, chopped
1 bay leaf
1 medium onion, sliced
½ tsp. ground turmeric
½ tsp. chili powder
1tsp. garam masala
1-inch cinnamon stick
1 tsp. crushed coriander seeds
1 tsp. ginger root, grated
1 tsp. garlic, crushed
½ tsp. salt
6 cups water

Heat oil in large frying pan or wok. Lower heat and add cloves, onion, peppercorn, and bay leaf. Cook for five minutes or until onion is golden brown. Add venison, turmeric, chili powder, garam masala, coriander seeds, garlic, ginger, cinnamon stick, and salt. Stir fry for about five minutes over medium heat. Add 3 ¾ cups of water and cover pan with lid. Simmer for about thirty-five to forty minutes, until water is evaporated.

Meanwhile, boil 2 ¼ cups of water in a small pot and add lentils. Boil for about ten to twelve minutes, until lentils are soft. Add lentils to venison stir-fry and mix well. Add tomatoes, chopped coriander and chilies to serve.

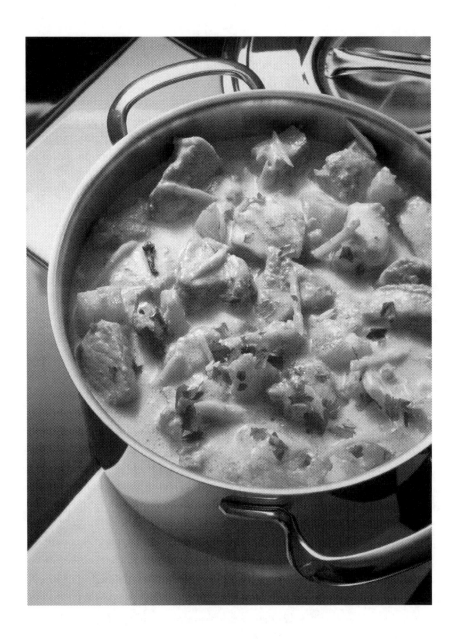

Lamb Chop Kashmiri
Serves 4

Ingredients:

8 to 12 lamb chops, about 3 ounces each
3 green cardamom pods
1 bay leaf
½ tsp. fennel seeds
A piece cinnamon bark
½ tsp. black peppercorns
1 tsp. salt
1 tsp. chili powder
1 ¼ cups corn oil
2 ½ cups milk
2/3 cup evaporated milk
2/3 cup plain yogurt
2 tbsp. all-purpose flour
1 tsp. ginger root, grated
1 tsp. chili powder
½ tsp. garlic, crushed
½ tsp. garam masala
1 ¼ cups corn oil
Pinch of salt
Mint sprigs
Lime quarters

Trim lamb chops and place in large pan. Add bay leaf, cinnamon bark, peppercorns, fennel seeds, and salt. Pour in milk and bring to a boil over high heat. Lower heat and cook for twelve to fifteen minutes or until milk has reduced to half. Next, pour in evaporated milk and lower heat to low. Simmer until lamb is completely cooked and milk has evaporated.

Meanwhile, blend yogurt, flour, chili powder, ginger, garam masala, crushed garlic, and salt in a large bowl. Remove chops from pan and add to yogurt mixture. Pan fry in a hot wok or deep skillet until chops are golden brown, turning once. Garnish with mint and lime quarters and serve immediately.

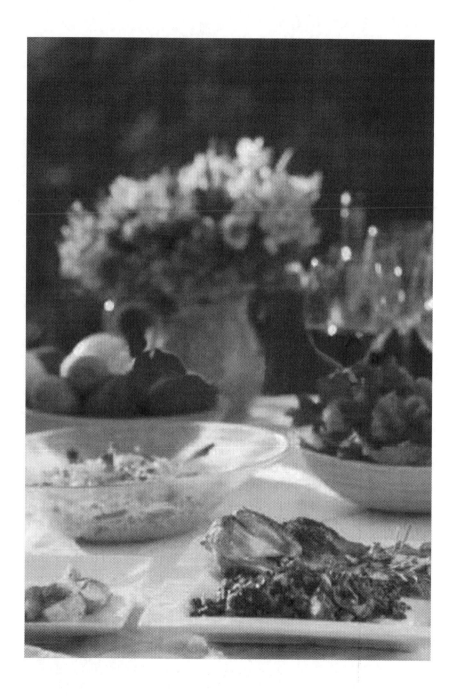

Saag Gosht
Lamb with Spinach
Serves 4–6

Ingredients:

1 ½ pounds lean lamb, cubed
1 tsp. garlic, crushed
1 tsp. garam masala
2 medium onions, sliced
1 tsp. ginger root, grated
1tsp. salt
1 1/2 tsp. chili powder
6 tbsp. corn oil
3 cups water
1 red bell pepper, chopped
3 green chilies, chopped
3 tbsp. coriander, chopped
14 ounces fresh spinach
1 tbsp. lemon juice

Mix together ginger, garlic, chili powder, salt, and garam masala. Set aside.

Heat oil in medium pan and fry onion until browned. Add lamb and fry for two minutes, stirring often. Next, add spice mixture and stir well. Pour in water and bring to a boil. Cover and lower heat, cooking for thirty minutes, or until water is evaporated.

Meanwhile, chop spinach roughly and blanch for about one minute. Drain well. Add spinach to the lamb when the water is evaporated. Fry over medium heat for eight minutes, stirring well. Add red pepper, green chilies, and coriander and stir over medium heat for two minutes. Sprinkle on lemon juice and serve immediately.

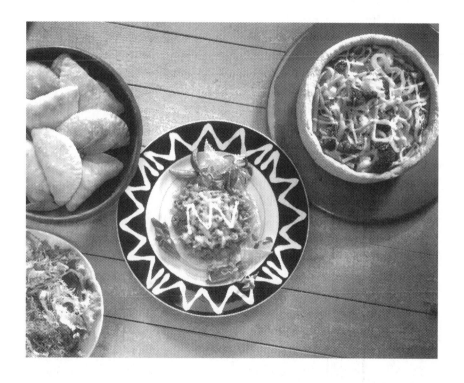

Lamb Dopiazza
Serves 4

Ingredients:

8 ounces lean lamb, cut into strips
1 tbsp. oil
8 baby onions
1 tsp. chili powder
1 tbsp. lemon juice
1tsp. ground cumin
1 tsp. ground coriander
1 tsp. salt
½ tsp. onion seeds
1 tbsp. lemon juice
4 curry leaves
1 green bell pepper, sliced
1 red bell pepper, sliced
1 ¼ cups water
1 tbsp. fresh mint
1 tbsp. fresh coriander

In a large bowl, mix together lamb, cumin, coriander, tomato puree, chili powder, salt, and lemon juice. Set aside. Heat oil in large wok or deep pan and stir fry the onion for about three minutes. Remove onion and set aside. Stir-fry onion seed and curry leaves in same pan for two to three minutes. Add the lamb and spice mixture and fry for five minutes. Pour in water, lower heat, and cook gently for ten minutes or until the lamb is cooked through. Add peppers and half of the coriander and mint. Cook another two minutes and then add the onion and remaining coriander and mint. Serve with rice.

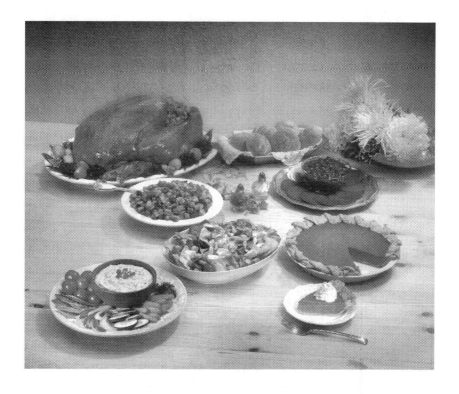

Malaysian Spicy Chicken
Serves 4

Ingredients:

1 pound boneless chicken, cubed
1 medium green mango
¼ tsp. onion seeds
1 tsp. ginger root, grated
½ tsp. garlic, crushed
1 tsp. chili powder
¼ tsp. ground turmeric
1 tsp. salt
2 tbsp. oil
1 tsp. ground coriander
2 onions, sliced
4 curry leaves
1 ¼ cups water
2 tomatoes, quartered
2 green chilies, chopped
2 tbsp. fresh coriander, chopped

Peel mango and slice into chunks. Place in a small bowl, cover, and set aside. In a large bowl, mix chicken, onion seeds, ginger, garlic, chili powder, turmeric, salt, coriander, and half the mango slices.

Heat oil in a medium pan and fry onion slices until brown. Add curry leaves and stir. Slowly add the chicken mixture, stirring constantly. Pour in water, lower heat, and simmer twelve to fifteen minutes until chicken is cooked and water is evaporated. Add tomatoes, remaining mango slices, green chilies, and coriander and serve hot.

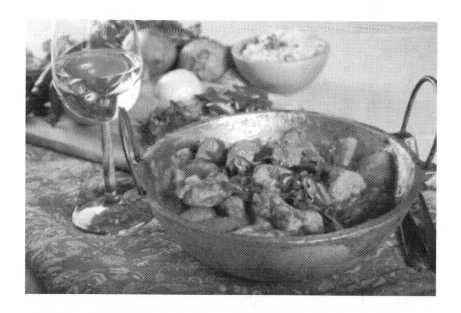

Spicy Chicken Curry
Serves 4

Ingredients:

12 ounces chicken, cubed
2 onions, chopped
½ red bell pepper, chopped
½ green bell pepper, chopped
2 tbsp. oil
¼ tsp. fenugreek seeds
¼ tsp. onion seeds
½ tsp. garlic, crushed
½ tsp. ginger root, grated
1 tsp. ground coriander
1 tsp. chili powder
1 tsp. salt
14 ounces canned tomatoes
2 tbsp. lemon juice
2 tbsp. fresh coriander
3 green chilies, chopped
Fresh coriander, to garnish

In a medium pan, heat oil and fry fenugreek and onion seeds until they become dark. Add chopped onions, garlic, and ginger. Fry about five minutes until the onions soften. Reduce heat to low.

Mix ground coriander, chili powder, salt, canned tomatoes, and lemon juice in a large bowl and stir well. Pour this mixture into pan and heat to medium. Fry about three minutes. Add chicken cubes and fry five to seven minutes. Then add fresh coriander, green chilies, and red and green bell peppers. Cover and lower heat, simmering for ten minutes until chicken is cooked. Serve the curry hot, garnished with fresh coriander.

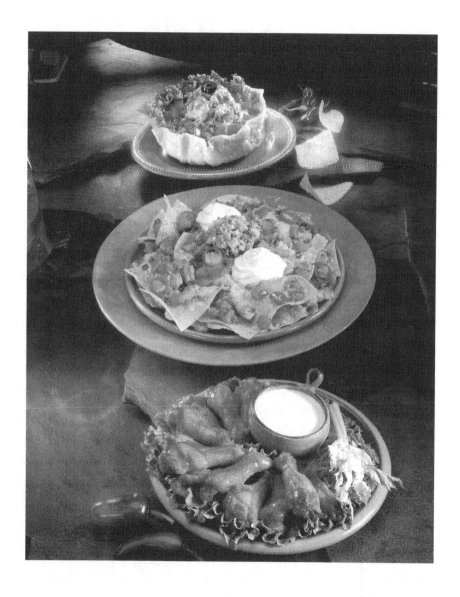

Karachi Chicken with Vegetables
Serves 4–6

Ingredients:

1 pound chicken breast, cut into strips
4 tbsp. corn oil
2 medium onions, sliced
4 garlic cloves, thickly sliced
1 tsp. salt
2 tbsp. lime juice
3 green chilies, chopped
2 medium carrots, sliced into medallions
2 medium potatoes, peeled and cut into strips
1 zucchini, sliced into medallions
4 lime slices
1 tbsp. coriander
2 green chilies, cut into strips

Heat oil in large wok or skillet and cook onions until browned. Add half the garlic, chicken, and salt. Cook everything together, stirring until chicken is lightly browned. Add lime juice, green chilies, and vegetables to the pan. Stir-fry for seven to ten minutes or until chicken is cooked through and the vegetables are tender. Garnish with lime juice, coriander, and green chilies. Serve immediately.

Chicken Biryani
Serves 4

Ingredients:

4 chicken breast fillets, cubed
1 1/2 cups basmati rice
10 whole green cardamom pods
2-inch cinnamon sticks
2–3 whole cloves
1/2 tsp salt
1/4 tsp hot chili powder
3 onions, sliced
3 tbsp. vegetable oil
1 tsp. ground coriander
1 tsp. ground cumin
3 garlic cloves, chopped
1/2 tsp. ground black pepper
1 tsp. finely chopped ginger root juice of one lemon
4 tomatoes, sliced
2 tbsp. fresh coriander, chopped
2/3 cup plain yogurt
4–5 saffron threads, soaked in 2 tsp. warm milk
2/3 cup water toasted almonds and fresh coriander, to garnish

Preheat oven to 375 degrees. Wash the rice and soak in water for thirty minutes. Remove seeds from cardamom pods and grind them finely, using a mortar and pestle. Set aside.

Next, bring a pan of water to a boil. Drain rice and add it to pan, with the salt, cardamom pods, cloves, and cinnamon stick. Boil for two minutes and then drain, leaving the spices in the rice. Cover rice and set aside. Heat oil in a large pan or wok and fry the onions for eight minutes, until softened. Now add the chicken and ground spices, including cardamom seeds. Mix well, and then add garlic, ginger, and lemon juice. Stir-fry for about five minutes and then transfer chicken mixture to a casserole pan.

Place tomatoes on top and garnish with the chopped coriander. Spoon the yogurt evenly across the casserole and then cover with rice. Drizzle the saffron milk over the rice and add water. Cover and bake for one hour. Transfer to a serving platter and discard the whole spices. Garnish with almond and coriander sprigs. Serve immediately.

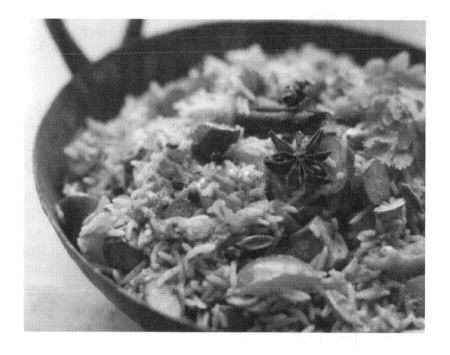

Masoor Biryani
Serves 4

Ingredients:

3/4 cup red split lentils
1 large potato
1/2 cup basmati rice
1 large onion, sliced
2 tbsp. oil
4 whole cloves
1/4 tsp. cumin seeds
1/4 tsp. ground turmeric
2 tsp. salt
1 1/4 cups water

Wash the lentils and rice in several changes of cold water and soak for fifteen minutes. Drain well and set aside. Heat oil in large pan and fry cloves and cumin seeds for two minutes until they begin to sputter. Peel and dice the potato and slice the onion. Add potato and onion to pan and fry for five minutes. Add lentils, rice, turmeric, and salt and cook for another three minutes. Add the water and bring mixture to a boil. Lower heat, cover and simmer for twenty minutes or until all the water evaporates and the potato is soft. Cover and let stand ten minutes before serving.

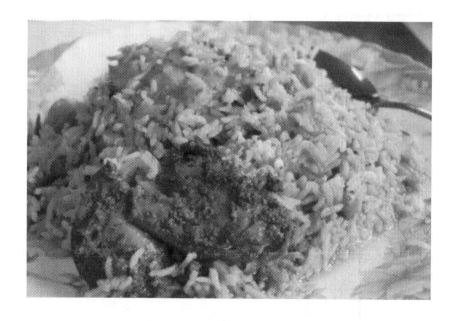

Gujrati Biryani
Serves 4–6

Ingredients:

1 cup long grain rice, washed seeds from 2 cardamom pods
2 whole cloves
2 garlic cloves
2 cups vegetable stock or broth
1 onion, chopped
1 tsp. cumin seeds
1 tsp. ground coriander
1/2 tsp. ground turmeric
1/2 tsp. chili powder
1 large potato, diced
2 carrots, sliced
1/2 cauliflower, broken into florets
2 ounces green beans, cut into one-inch lengths
2 tbsp. fresh coriander, chopped
2 tbsp. lime juice salt and pepper

Preheat oven to 350 degrees. In a large, heavy pan, add rice, cloves, cardamom seeds, and vegetable stock. Bring to a rolling boil and then cover and reduce heat. Simmer for twenty minutes or until stock has been absorbed. Meanwhile, place garlic cloves, onion, cumin seeds, ground coriander, turmeric, chili powder, and salt and pepper in a blender or food processor with two tablespoons of water. Blend until smooth. Put the paste in a large casserole dish and place over a low heat for two minutes, stirring occasionally. Next add potato, carrots, cauliflower, and beans, along with four tablespoons of water. Cover mixture and cook over a low heat for twelve minutes, stirring occasionally. Add the fresh chopped coriander. Remove the cloves from the rice and discard. Add rice to the vegetable mixture and sprinkle with lime juice. Cover and place in the over for twenty-five minutes or until all the vegetables are tender. Fluff rice and garnish with fresh coriander before serving.

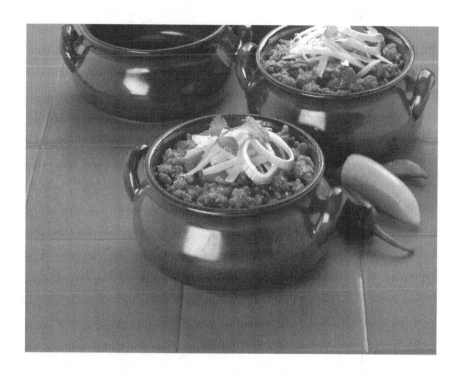

Fava Gobhi
Serves 4

Ingredients:

1 garlic cloves, chopped
1-inch piece fresh ginger root
1 green chili, seeded and chopped
2 tbsp. oil
1 onion, sliced
1 large potato, diced
1 tbsp. curry powder, mild or hot cauliflower, cut into small florets
2 1/2 cups vegetable stock or broth
10-ounce can of fava beans juice of 1/2 a lemon salt and pepper fresh coriander sprig, to garnish plain rice, to serve

Blend garlic, ginger, chili, and one tablespoon of oil in a food processor or blender until smooth. Set aside. In a large pan, fry potato and onion in one tablespoon of oil for five minutes, and then add the spice paste and curry powder. Cook for one more minute, and then add cauliflower and stir well. Next, add the vegetable stock and bring the mixture to a rolling boil over high heat. Add salt and pepper and then cover and simmer for ten minutes. Now add the fava beans, including the liquid in the can. Cook uncovered for another ten minutes. Sprinkle lemon juice on mixture and add salt and pepper to taste. Garnish with fresh coriander and serve with plain rice.

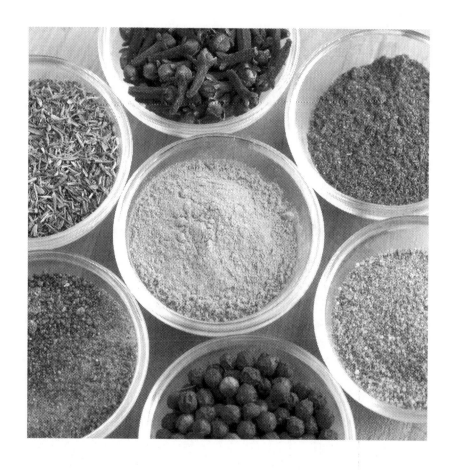

Spicy Karahi Aloo
Serves 4

Ingredients:

6 waxy potatoes, thinly sliced
1 tbsp. oil
1 tsp. cumin seeds
1 tsp. crushed dried red chilies
1 red chili, seeded and sliced
1 green chili, seeded and sliced
3 curry leaves
1/2 tsp. mixed onion, mustard, and fenugreek seeds
1/2 tsp. fennel seeds
3 garlic cloves, sliced
1-inch piece ginger root, grated
2 onions, sliced
1 tbsp. fresh coriander, chopped

Heat oil in large pan or wok and add cumin seeds, curry leaves, dried red chilies, mixed onion, fenugreek, and mustard seeds, fennel seeds, garlic, and ginger. Fry for one minute, and then add onion and fry for another five minutes or until the onions have softened. Next, add the potatoes, fresh coriander, and red and green chilies. Mix well and cover, cooking for seven minutes on low heat or until potatoes are tender. Serve hot straight from pan.

Conclusion

As I recalled earlier, I have been a devotee of Shaolin Kung Fu since a very young age. Something instilled in that practice applies perhaps even more so to our physical health. "This is not a hobby, this is a lifestyle; if you live it, then you will be it," was the mantra told over and over again to me by my teacher. And that mantra has been my life's inspiration. More importantly, I feel it applies to everything you have learned in this book as well. For both myself (working as a physical trainer) and my partner, Dr. Noor (with his patients), we have never once told anyone to "lose weight." Instead, we have stressed the importance of making gradual (but profound) lifestyle changes. This philosophy gets at the heart of what the *Desi Diet* truly is, and I sincerely hope that you have already found the power inherent in this method.

The *Desi Diet* Is a Lifestyle, Not a Diet

And that's a good thing, actually, because as we discussed earlier, the vast majority of diets, nearly 95 percent according to most studies, *simply do not work.* Instead, most dieters actually go on to gain weight once their diet period is over. As we have shown earlier, our bodies are genetically hardwired to gain weight. From our prehistoric days when early humans were hunters and gatherers, until as recently as our agricultural society (which, outside of America, is still the predominant system across much of the globe), when food is scarce, our bodies are actually programmed to gain weight. When our body doesn't get the proper food it needs, it automatically thinks that we were going into starvation mode, preparing for a long, cold winter, and so on. So diets, then, actually "trick" the body into believing that it is going into a period of fasting, and the body reacts by conserving fat and burning muscle—exactly the opposite of what any proper health regimen should do.

That's why we have designed the *Desi Diet* (yes, despite its unforgettable, slightly misleading name) to be a profound lifestyle change, and not a diet. In summary, it includes:

- Differentiating between good and bad carbs
- The importance of getting on a good vitamin/supplement routine
- Water and its absolute importance in any proper health program
- Considering—not obsessing over—calories
- Tapering meal size
- The supreme importance of getting enough good sleep
- How to better manage stress
- Great recipe and meal ideas
- The proper cooking methods: good and bad fats
- And much, much more . . .

Get Ready for . . . More Energy!

By learning to eat the right foods—whole, unprocessed ones—and in quantities that exceed your resting metabolic rate, you will undergo steady and sustained weight loss. This will help you get off the yo-yo, seesaw trend of "fad" diets. The results your body will feel will be nothing short of staggering. As you begin to eliminate the unhealthy fats, overload of sugars, and plethora of chemicals found in much of your traditional diet, your body will unleash a sustained, high level of energy that you may not have experienced in years.

The Best Part of the *Desi Diet*: Reducing or Eliminating Medications

As cited earlier, the Desi community, unfortunately, has an incredibly high incidence of risk factors for coronary artery disease (CAD), including insulin resistance, diabetes, a high lipid profile, a generally sedentary lifestyle, and increased, sustained levels of stress. But this does not mean there is nothing we can do about it.

Following the recommendations in the *Desi Diet* will help you succeed in not only your weight loss but also your long-term health and well-being. Remember that food speaks to our genes. Turning on the "right" ones and minimizing the impact of the "negative" ones are key in resisting disease, losing a range of chronic symptoms, and creating optimal health—which means getting off medications sooner, rather than later,. It is important to remember that *all* medications have some side effects. Antibiotics, which are now readily handed out for everything from pneumonia to serious chronic illnesses, have a wide range of side effects—and in fact, many diseases/bacteria have built up resistance to them. Blood-thinning medicines, often prescribed to the elderly or those with heart/circulation disorders, can cause dire consequences if the prescribed individual develops a laceration and does not properly form clots. Even a medicine as "safe" and common as Tylenol can destroy your liver if you take too much of it.

How the Desi Diet Will Boost Your Self-Confidence and Self-Esteem

Taking control of your diet and watching the pounds melt off can mean a lot of things to different people, from the way they look in the mirror and see a different person to the warm feelings that come with compliments they receive from their loved ones. It can be as simple as the way they can now fit into a pair of jeans they haven't worn in years. Or perhaps most importantly, just the quiet confidence that comes with knowing they will be around longer for their loved ones.

Setting and Hitting Goals—without Getting Sidetracked

When most people decide to lose weight or change their lifestyle, they tend to make the mistake of setting overly tough goals—such as losing a tremendous amount of weight at once. Just setting one large goal—without filling in the dots and creating an actual action plan to get you there—will almost guarantee that you get easily discouraged by setbacks and lose all motivation. Undoubtedly, frustration can then set in. This one large goal becomes too much, and you may give up altogether.

Instead, if you can create a clear idea of exactly what you want to accomplish—again, a notebook or journal to record your plans will serve well here—you will then naturally set smaller, short term health goals that are more specific to your needs. (Think, "I want cut down my sugar intake this week, and begin walking every day," as opposed to, "I need to lose seventy-five pounds now!"). Smaller goals will be more reachable, more realistic, and in most cases, nothing short of empowering!

And as you reach your first goal, be sure to look to set your sights on a new and more challenging one.

The Importance of Taking Gradual Steps

Remember to never overdo it when it comes to a new fitness or health regime. Always consult your physician before beginning a new exercise program and/or implementing a change in diet, especially if you are new to exercise, injury-prone, or have some other chronic health condition.

When setting goals—regarding health, fitness, or dietary changes—learn to recognize your current limitations, and set your short-term goals accordingly. Yes, you can challenge yourself but not to the point of injury or a bruised self-confidence. (In fact, I have seen this scenario unfold many times in the gym where I train others.)

How to Stay on Track

Once you have reached your desired body composition—and I trust that after reading the *Desi Diet* you may be well along your way—don't go back to bad habits. Whatever the bad habit(s) were that got you out of shape in the first place, try to avoid them when you feel the urge. Whether that was eating immediately before you go to bed, loading up on sugars, or leading a sedentary lifestyle, if you feel those old habits creeping back, recognize them and try to find activities to take their place.

Actually, the good news is that *it will actually be hard to develop new bad habits.* The power of the *Desi Diet* is that it will boost your confidence and energy and cut your reliance on all the unhealthy foods that used to be such a part of your life.

Staying Positive and Finding Support

The hardest part of any endeavor is finding support. So as you change your lifestyle, don't be afraid to ask for help when you need it. Whether it's from your spouse or family, physician or healthcare provider—or even your jogging or workout buddy—there is help there, if you ask. And the best part? Once you begin bettering yourself, you will be able to reflect a positive attitude for your friends and family and be a better person for them.

The Last Word: Spreading the News to Your Family and Loved Ones

Once you have reached your goals—or even if you are just beginning to reach your first small steps—it is important to consider spreading the word to your friends and family in reaching the same goal of living a healthy lifestyle. Some religions have long had a "conversion" element to them. Today, tech companies have "evangelists" who speak out about the benefits of the latest gadget or widget. We feel, as Desis, that we need to "speak out" about the importance of good health. We are tired of watching our parents' generation die of heart attacks and diabetes and cringe as we see our friends growing older and neglecting their health.

Today Desi culture has marched out onto the global stage and is serving as a role model for much of the world. But it is a shame when so many of our best and brightest are dying so young for no reason other than poor eating habits and no fitness plan. Sure, we can enjoy our occasional *roti, paratha*—and even *ghee.* But we shouldn't be letting those foods kill us in the process.

[1], ² http://www.southasianheartcenter.org/

[2]

[3] www.who.org

BODY MASS INDEX TABLE

Check your heights in inches in the left column and your weight in pounds
in the corresponding right columns. Your BMI value will be at the bottom of
the column of your weight

		W	E	I	G	H	T		I	N		P	O	U	N	D	S							
H	58	91	96	100	105	110	115	119	124	129	134	138	143	148	153	158	162	167	172	177	181	186	191	196
E	59	94	99	104	109	114	119	124	128	133	138	143	148	153	158	163	168	173	178	183	188	193	198	203
I	60	97	102	107	112	118	123	128	133	138	143	148	153	158	163	168	174	179	184	189	194	199	204	209
G	61	100	106	111	116	122	127	132	137	143	148	153	158	164	169	174	180	185	190	195	201	206	211	217
H	62	104	109	115	120	126	131	136	142	147	153	158	164	169	175	180	186	191	196	202	207	213	218	224
T	63	107	113	118	124	130	135	141	146	152	158	163	169	175	180	186	191	197	203	208	214	220	225	231
	64	110	116	122	128	134	140	145	151	157	163	169	174	180	186	192	197	204	209	215	221	227	232	238
I	65	114	120	126	132	138	144	150	156	162	168	174	180	186	192	198	204	210	216	222	228	234	240	246
N	66	118	124	130	136	142	148	155	161	167	173	179	186	192	198	204	210	216	223	229	235	241	247	253
	67	121	127	134	140	146	153	159	166	172	178	185	191	198	204	211	217	223	230	236	242	249	255	261
I	68	125	131	138	144	151	158	164	171	177	184	190	197	203	210	216	223	230	236	243	249	256	262	269
N	69	128	135	142	149	155	162	169	176	182	189	196	203	209	216	223	230	236	243	250	257	263	270	277
C	70	132	139	146	153	160	167	174	181	188	195	202	209	216	222	229	236	243	250	257	264	271	278	285
H	71	136	143	150	157	165	172	179	186	193	200	208	215	222	229	236	243	250	257	265	272	279	286	293
E	72	140	147	154	162	169	177	184	191	199	206	213	221	228	235	242	250	258	265	272	279	287	294	302
S	73	144	151	159	166	174	182	189	197	204	212	219	227	235	242	250	257	265	272	280	288	295	302	310
	74	148	155	163	171	179	186	194	202	210	218	225	233	241	249	256	264	272	280	287	295	303	311	319
	75	152	160	168	176	184	192	200	208	216	224	232	240	248	256	264	272	279	287	295	303	311	319	327
	76	159	164	172	180	189	197	205	213	221	230	238	246	254	263	271	279	287	295	304	312	320	328	336
BMI		19	20	21	22	23	24	25	26	27	28	29	30	31	32	33	34	35	36	37	38	39	40	41

BMI Values   Below 25   Normal
                     25 to 29   Overweight
                     30 to 39   Obese
                     40 and up   Extreme Obesity